Goddesses Don't Diet

THE GIRLFRIENDS' GUIDE TO
INTERMITTENT FASTING

Yvonne Aileen

800 Muses Publishing

PORTLAND, OREGON

800MUSES.com

FDA Disclaimer

The information contained herein has not been evaluated by the Food & Drug Administration or any other medical body. Neither the author nor publisher claim to diagnose, treat, cure, or prevent any illness or disease. Information is shared for educational purposes only. The content of this book is not intended to be a substitute for professional medical advice, diagnosis, or treatment. Do not disregard or delay obtaining medical advice for any medical condition you may have and seek the assistance of your health care professional for any such conditions.

Consult your doctor before acting on any content herein, especially if you are pregnant, nursing, taking medication, or have a medical condition.

Copyright © 2021 by Yvonne Aileen.

All rights reserved. No part of this publication may be reproduced, distributed, or transmitted in any form or by any means, including photocopying, recording, or other electronic or mechanical methods, without the prior written permission of the publisher, except in the case of brief quotations embodied in critical reviews and certain other noncommercial uses permitted by copyright law.

For permission requests, write to the publisher, subject line: "Attention: Permissions Coordinator," at the address below.

publisher@800Muses.com
www.800Muses.com

Ordering Information:

Quantity sales. Special discounts are available on quantity purchases by corporations, associations, and others. For details, contact the "Special Sales Department" at the address above.

GODDESSES DON'T DIET: THE GIRLFRIENDS' GUIDE TO INTERMITTENT FASTING / Yvonne Aileen. —1st ed.

ISBN 978-1-7369105-1-1

Contents

Golly! 1
The Obesity-Diabetes Connection 5
Dieting: The Big Fat Lie 9
You've Got A Friend in Fung 36
IF, OMAD, ADF, WTF? 50
Are You Ready? Why Timing Is Crucial to Success 69
The Keto Connection 75
Help for Carb and Sugar Addicts 79
Sleep, Water, and Exercise 89
The Climacteric Conundrum 106
Anti-Aging and IF 111
Fast Drivers 115
Food Dreams and Flashcards: My 14-Day Fast 133
Goddess in the Kitchen: Recipes and Pantry Items 147
Expect Resistance 160
Affirmations for Your Intermittent Fasting Journey 163
Acknowledgments 169
To You, Goddess 171
For Further Reading 172
About the Author 175

*To the captains of commerce in the weight loss industry
who see our desperation and desire as dollar signs,
who build their wealth at the expense of our health—
up yours.*

*If diets actually worked,
we wouldn't have to go on so many of them.*

— Psychologist Alexis Conason
New York Obesity Nutrition Research Center

Never go on another diet again.

Dear Goddess

I'm not a doctor, and nothing in here should be construed as medical advice. There are lots of great books available on intermittent fasting and its many health and weight loss benefits. *The Girlfriends' Guide to Intermittent Fasting will point you to some of these. Together, we'll get into the science a bit, but let's leave most of that for the white coats. Instead, I want to share with you the real-world, in-the-trenches, messy truth, in the same way I would with a girlfriend. This includes my struggle with weight and health issues, the bonehead mistakes I've made, and how I was able to finally get off the diet hamster wheel once and for all.*

Why didn't anyone tell us all this before?

Because there was no money in it.

Yvonne

INTRODUCTION

Golly!

ON MAUI'S SOUTH SIDE is the town of Kihei, where the people who can't afford to buy or rent in tonier Wailea live. Kihei is a mixture of time-shares, vacation rentals, and modest but expensive homes, as well as shave ice stalls, canoe clubs, surfboard rentals, and all the shops and restaurants you'd expect in a resort town. As a transplant from Oregon with a modest income, I had purchased a condo in the *north* part of Kihei, where the people who can't afford to buy or rent on Kihei's *south* side live. Some call north Kihei *Ki-hell* because it's dustier and hotter than the south side. To me, it was affordable paradise.

I had been there a little more than a year when I made an appointment with a naturopath.

"I think something's wrong with me," I told the George Hamilton look-alike. "I exercise and eat lightly, and I still can't lose weight."

"George" gave me a heard-it-all-before movie star smile. "You're probably low on estrogen, like most women your age." He then recommended synthetic hormone replacement therapy and pointed to a shelf in his office that had row upon row of white boxes with what I assume contained the magic cure. I told him I didn't want pharmaceuticals; I just wanted a body like Jennifer Aniston's. Was that too much to ask?

He ordered lab tests. On this, my second visit, he shared the results. "Your estrogen levels are a little low, and you're prediabetic."

"What does *pre*diabetic mean?" I flashed back to another doctor visit, 20 years earlier on the mainland when my doctor told me that my pap smear showed that my cervix had *pre*cancerous cells. *Precancerous* cells, she explained, were somewhere on the continuum between normal cells and cancer cells. So, according to the naturopath, I was on the continuum between not being diabetic and *being* diabetic.

"What do I need to do?"

"Watch your diet," was his only advice as he glanced regretfully at the magic boxes.

Although it beat the heck out of a cone biopsy, "watch your diet" didn't give me a lot to go on. What woman didn't *already* watch her diet?

So, nothing changed after that. I didn't overindulge in sugar, but I never had. And I had always eaten healthy (or so I thought), so I mostly tried to ignore what I'd learned in the naturopath's office, reasoning that if it were serious, George would have said so.

As the years passed, in darker moments, I did occasionally think about a former neighbor of my in-laws. I don't remember her name, but she had a lumbering way of walking that reminded me of Mrs. Golly from *Harriet the Spy*. This Mrs. Golly often needed rides to the doctor and sometimes to the hospital where she would lose another body part. "Sugar diabetes," my mother-in-law had explained.

Although hearing about those hospital visits made me shudder, sugar diabetes was far removed from my reality—from *any* reality, for that matter, sounding like something fairies bestowed on good children—not something that would cause you to lose your toes, your feet, and eventually, your life.

I later learned that *sugar diabetes* is an old-fashioned term for type 2 diabetes. And Mrs. Golly had it, until it had her. She'd been a hoarder as well. When they cleared out her house, they found cupboards stacked with thousands of plastic containers from previously consumed TV dinners. Perversely, I was relieved by that discovery. "Sugar diabetes will never happen to me," I thought. "I don't eat that crap."

And now here I was, pre-Golly.

CHAPTER 1

The Obesity-Diabetes Connection

IT'S HARD TO CHASE THE NUMBERS. It's still commonly said that "more than a third" of adults in the United States are obese. But figures released in February 2021 by the Centers for Disease Control (CDC) report that the prevalence of obesity in the US had climbed to 42.4%. Although technically "more than a third," that number is 10 points higher than it was 20 years ago.[1] Worldwide obesity rates have tripled since 1975. Currently, most of the world lives in countries where being overweight or obese kills more people than being malnourished and underweight.[2]

In Europe, the UK has the highest level of obesity. The majority of adults are overweight or obese; 67% of men and 60% of women are

---

[1] "Adult Diabetes Facts," CDC.gov (May 25, 2021) https://www.cdc.gov/obesity/data/adult.html
[2] "Obesity and overweight," World Health Organization (April 1, 2020) https://www.who.int/news-room/fact-sheets/detail/obesity-and-overweight

overweight and 26% of men and 29% of women in the UK are obese.[3] The Pacific Islands and Middle East nations have even higher rates than the US and UK.

Obesity and type 2 diabetes are inextricably linked. In fact, obesity is the best predictor of whether a person will develop type 2 diabetes. Even being overweight can increase your chances of developing type 2 diabetes. And according to the CDC, one in five people in the US who has diabetes doesn't know it.[4] And prediabetes? *Fuhgettaboutit.* More than one in three Americans has prediabetes, and 84% of those with the disease don't know they have it.[5] Per the CDC:

> Prediabetes is a serious health condition where blood sugar levels are higher than normal, but not high enough yet to be diagnosed as type 2 diabetes.
>
> Prediabetes is diagnosed through blood glucose testing after an overnight fast. A level between 100 and 125 mg/dL indicates prediabetes. A level of 126 mg/dL indicates type 2 diabetes.

---

[3] "Statistics on Obesity, Physical Activity and Diet," National Health Service (May 5, 2020) https://digital.nhs.uk/data-and-information/publications/statistical/statistics-on-obesity-physical-activity-and-diet/england-2020

[4] "Diabetes Fast Facts," CDC.gov (May 25, 2021) https://www.cdc.gov/diabetes/basics/quick-facts.html

[5] "Prediabetes – Your Chance to Prevent Type 2 Diabetes," CDC.gov (May 25, 2021) https://www.cdc.gov/diabetes/basics/prediabetes.html

Are You Prediabetic?

Do you have prediabetes? Would you know? The only way to know for sure is to measure your blood sugar level. Prediabetes is not something to be taken lightly. Per the Mayo Clinic, "... the long-term damage of diabetes—especially to your heart, blood vessels, and kidneys—may already be starting" at the prediabetes stage. There are usually no signs or symptoms, but one possible indication is darkened skin on the neck, armpits, elbows, knees, or knuckles.[6] Per the Mayo Clinic, symptoms that indicate you've graduated from "pre" to full-blown type 2 diabetes are:

- Increased thirst
- Frequent urination
- Excess hunger
- Blurred vision
- Fatigue

"Diabetes – the physical costs: Hypertension: 70% of diabetics also require medication for blood pressure. Cholesterol: 65% of diabetics require medication to reduce their cholesterol. Heart attacks: Diabetics, even when on full medication, are twice as likely to be hospitalised, crippled or die from a heart attack. Strokes: Diabetics are 1.5 times more likely to suffer a debilitating stroke. Blindness and Eye Problems: Diabetes is the number one cause of preventable blindness in the developed world.

---

[6] "Prediabetes" Mayo Clinic (May 25, 2021) https://www.mayoclinic.org/diseases-conditions/prediabetes/symptoms-causes/syc-20355278

Impotence: Diabetes is also the number one cause of impotence. Dementia: Having diabetes doubles your risk of dementia. Kidney disease: Diabetes is the cause of kidney failure in half of all new cases; most people on dialysis are diabetics."

— **Michael Mosley,** *The 8-week Blood Sugar Diet: Lose Weight Fast and Reprogramme Your Body*

"It's no coincidence, I think, that obesity rates began rising rapidly in the 1980s more or less in tandem with this widespread endorsement of more frequent meals."
— **Andrew Weil, MD,** *Eating Well for Optimum Health*

"According to the surgeon general, obesity today is officially an epidemic; it is arguably the most pressing public health problem we face, costing the health care system an estimated $90 billion a year.

Because of diabetes and all the other health problems that accompany obesity, today's children may turn out to be the first generation of Americans whose life expectancy will actually be shorter than that of their parents.

The problem is not limited to America: The United Nations reported that in 2000 the number of people suffering from overnutrition—a billion—had officially surpassed the number suffering from malnutrition—800 million."
— **Michael Pollan,** *The Omnivore's Dilemma: A Natural History of Four Meals*

CHAPTER 2

Dieting: The Big Fat Lie

PABLO PICASSO, a brilliant artist and a notorious cad, once informed his mistress, "For me, there are only two kinds of women: goddesses and doormats." He was wrong. Every woman is a goddess, even when—for the sake of penises or profits—others treat us like doormats.

We have been lied to for decades. Once women reach perimenopause (and certainly beyond menopause), the weight loss game is stacked against us, and the old rules no longer apply. When I was in my twenties, if I gained a few pounds, all I had to do was pick up a two-week supply of SlimFast, replace two meals a day, and like magic, the pounds vanished into thinner air. In my 40s, after having two children, I gained some weight. Some? The Special K model couldn't pinch an inch. I could grab a slab.

I repeated my no-fail SlimFast method, filling my grocery cart with several packs of Dark Chocolate Fudge, already tasting victory. I followed the plan faithfully for the usual two weeks and then stepped on the scale triumphantly. But I had only lost one pound! "SlimFast must have changed its formula!" I thought.

So, I tried Weight Watchers and Jenny Craig and Nutrisystem and the Lemonade Diet and the Cabbage Soup Diet and LA Weight Loss and the General Motors Diet. I became a consumer of (and rep for) Isagenix products. I injected myself with hCG (human chorionic gonadotropin) and cut back to 500 calories a day. I signed up for Spark People and got a pedometer and logged 10,000 steps every day for months. I bought exercise videos and did Buns of Steel and 8-Minute Abs and the 30-Day Shred, committing myself to two workouts a day. On a hiking trip to Sedona, Arizona, I was more than a little smug that my two hiking companions, who were 10 and 20 years younger than me, had trouble keeping up due to foot and knee injuries. Pride goeth before the fall. Right after I returned from that trip, I bought special fitness shoes advertised to help me "use more muscle with every step." But after wearing them for five-mile walking workouts two days in a row, I woke up on Day 3 and could not put any weight on my left foot. That resulted in a recurring injury that has plagued me for years.

And after all of that, what were my results?
- I lost a few pounds.
- I experienced soul-killing plateaus.
- I regained what I'd lost and then some.

Every. Damned. Time.

As I struggled for all those years, one tiny consolation was that I wasn't alone. Among my friends and family members who were also "women of a certain age," most struggled with permanent weight loss, yo-yoing their way through one fad, one program, one miracle-cure-that-wasn't after another. Together and separately, we joined gyms and bought exercise equipment and workout clothes and supplements and endured cleanses and body wraps. We excitedly signed up for the latest diet program or plan, compared progress, and hoped that this time it would be different. Collectively, we were P.T. Barnum's sucker born every minute,[7] gasping for air on our yoga mats only to rise and do battle again the next day … the next week … the next month … the next year … and yes, the next decade. Our hard-won temporary successes always led to rapid backslides, as if we were climbing concrete mountains while wearing roller skates.

Dieting Is Big Business

Our battle of the bulge came with a legion of cheerleaders urging us back onto the battlefield. A $78B weight loss industry depended on us for its profits, and we did not disappoint. Segments of this industry we supported with our money, hope, and trust include:

- Weight loss programs
- Meal replacement products

---

[7] Legend has it that Barnum never said this; perhaps it was Jenny Craig.

- Diet pills
- Supplements
- Exercise videos and subscriptions
- Health clubs
- Slimming teas
- Frozen diet entrees
- Multi-level marketing channels
- Medical programs
- Diet books, DVDs, and apps
- Diet soft drinks
- Artificial sweeteners

These heavy hitters in this industry knew our names:

- WW (formerly Weight Watchers), 5 million members in 2020; 2019 sales of $1.4B[8]
- Jenny Craig, revenues of $400M (2018 figures)[9]
- Nutrisystem, $691M in revenue in 2018[10]

---

[8] "WW Announces Fourth Quarter and Full Year 2019 Results and Provides Full Year 2020 Guidance" Intrado Global Newswire (Feb. 5, 2020) https://www.globenewswire.com/news-release/2020/02/25/1990458/0/en/WW-Announces-Fourth-Quarter-and-Full-Year-2019-Results-and-Provides-Full-Year-2020-Guidance.html

[9] Mariel Concepcion, "Jenny Craig Puts Retail Presence Into Plan," *San Diego Business* Journal (Jan. 20, 2020) https://www.sdbj.com/news/2020/jan/20/jenny-craig-puts-retail-presence-plans/

[10] "Nutrisystem Announces Fourth Quarter and Full Year 2018 Financial Results," Business Wire (Feb 19, 2019) https://www.businesswire.com/news/home/20190219005700/en/Nutrisystem-Announces-Fourth-Quarter-and-Full-Year-2018-Financial-Results

- Herbalife, $1.2B in 2019[11] (weight management products deliver 61.8% of its revenue)
- Isagenix, $6B in global sales in 2018[12]
- Medifast, approximate sales of $1B in 2021

You probably recognize most of these names, but other key players in the weight loss and weight management industry include:

- Cargill[13]
- PepsiCo, Inc.
- Kellogg Company
- General Mills, Inc.
- Abbott, maker of Similac, PediaSure, Pedialyte, and Ensure
- The Kraft Heinz Company
- Ingredion[14]

Big Food and Big Pharma both have a stake in the weight loss and weight management industry. Their profits are dependent on keeping us dependent on their products.

---

[11] Emma Bedford, "Herbalife's net sales share worldwide in 2019, by product category," Statista (Sept 28, 2020) https://www.statista.com/statistics/917722/herbalife-net-sales-share-by-product-category-worldwide/

[12] "Isagenix Hits $6 Billion in Cumulative Global Sales," Isagenix (May 4, 2018) https://newsroom.isagenix.com/isagenix-hits-6-billion-in-cumulative-global-sales/

[13] With sales of $114.6B, Cargill is the largest privately held corporation in the US in terms of revenue. Purina® brand pet food is one of its product lines. In the weight loss channel, its brands include EverSweet and Stevia Sweetener.

[14] Manufacturer of the Best Foods brand, Skippy peanut butter, Knorr, Hellman's; producing mainly starch, modified starches and starch sugars such as glucose syrup and high fructose syrup.

What's in Those Meal Replacements?

Meal replacements come in the form of shakes and other prepared foods. Here are a few ingredients in some of the most popular meal replacements:

SlimFast

These shakes contain a variety of sweeteners, preservatives, food stabilizers, canola oil, and hydrogenated soybean oil. Most nutritionists recommend limiting hydrogenated soybean oil, given its potential negative effects on the body due to the trans fatty acids it produces.[15] They also contain a whopping 31 grams of carbs, 18 grams of sugar, and only 10 grams of protein.

Jenny Craig

When evaluating the list of ingredients in Jenny Craig meal replacements, nutritionists found that the healthiest part of the plan by far was the fresh food the consumer supplied. The company's prepared foods were high in refined sugars, far too low in fat, low in fiber, and too low in calories. They were also dominated by additives, artificial ingredients, added sugars, and hydrogenated oils (trans fat).[16] The Jenny Craig program is based on restricted calories, fat and portion control, and eating six times a day (three meals and

---

[15] Kaitlin Ahern, "How to Find the Weight-Loss Program That Will Work for You," Livestrong.com (Aug 8, 2019) https://www.livestrong.com/article/13720774-best-weight-loss-programs/

[16] Megan Steinrager, "Prepared Diet Food: The Good, the Bad, and the Unhealthy," Epicurious (May 25, 2021) https://www.epicurious.com/archive/healthy/news/dietdelivery_jennycraig

three snacks), which means multiple insulin spikes. We'll discuss why that's problematic later.

Nutrisystem

Nutritionists threw Nutrisystem similar shade, finding that about half of the calories from the plan (the most nutritious half consisting of dairy and protein, fresh fruits, and vegetables) came from foods the consumer is meant to provide. The heavily processed, shelf-stable (or for pricier plans, frozen) prepackaged food was found to contain a long list of artificial ingredients, synthetic nutrients, preservatives, and trans fats and contained very little fiber, calcium, antioxidants, or calories.[17]

Medifast

Ingredients include Medifast meal replacements include fructose, sugar, acesulfame potassium (more easily pronounced by its other name Ace-K), corn syrup solids, dextrose, and soy protein isolate.[18] Ace-K is an artificial sweetener that contains the carcinogen methylene chloride, and while studies aren't yet definitive, this ingredient has been linked to cancer.[19]

---

[17] Ibid; https://www.epicurious.com/archive/healthy/news/dietdelivery_nutrisystem

[18] Denise Webb, "Liquid Meal Replacements," Today's Dietitian, vol. 1, No. 1, p. 20 (January 2018 issue) https://www.todaysdietitian.com/newarchives/0118p20.shtml

[19] Anna Schaefer, "Is Acesulfame Potassium Bad for Me?" Healthline (Nov 10, 2017) https://www.healthline.com/health/is-acesulfame-potassium-bad-for-me#evidence-of-risks

Optifast

A Nestle product, Optifast meal replacements contain milk protein isolate, maltodextrin, canola oil, soy lecithin, sucralose, and artificial flavors. Here's what you eat on an Optifast diet, per its own website:

> *Dietary intake will consist of one OPTIFAST VLCD [very low-calorie diet] Product, two low calorie meals (approximately 400 calories each), at least two cups of low starch vegetables, two serves [sic] of fruit, one serve [sic] of dairy and two liters of water.*[20]

My former crush on SlimFast notwithstanding, I have a deep loathing of liquid meal replacements because I believe they were a contributing factor in the death of my mother.

In her 30s, after having five children and experiencing some serious medical issues, my mother gained weight and eventually became obese. She tried many methods to lose the weight. Several years prior to her death, she went on a drastic "medically supervised" very low-calorie diet consisting of a powdered drink mix and very little else. I learned of this when she came to visit me for my college graduation, and I noticed her in my kitchen mixing up this concoction in a specially made shaker cup.

She'd lost considerable weight, but I'd never seen her look so unhealthy. Her cheeks were sunken, her skin pale, and her hair was

---

[20] "Optifast VLCD Program Weight Loss Phases," Nestle Health Science (May 25, 2021) https://www.nestlehealthscience-me.com/en/health-management/obesity/optifast-vlcd-programme

falling out. Later, she confided to me that she was often so constipated that she had to use extraordinary means to eliminate.

Once my mother was off the program, her weight came back, and she became heavier than ever. Years later, she was diagnosed with stage IV colon cancer. Colon cancer is easily detectable if you get a colonoscopy (she hadn't), and it can take 10 to 15 years to develop into cancer. This would have coincided with her meal replacement period. I believe there was another contributing factor to my mother's death: embarrassment. My mother didn't go to a doctor for screening because she was embarrassed about her weight. She died at age 59 from complications related to her chemotherapy treatment post-surgery.

In addition to being less than optimally nutritious and comparatively expensive, long-term success rates for meal replacement products are abysmal. They don't teach portion control, they offer low-calorie, carb-laden, unhealthy food options, and when consumers stop relying on them for meal replacement, they're often at a loss to know what to eat. So, the weight comes back on, making all that deprivation pointless—worse than pointless—*injurious* to their health.

Frozen Meals

As an alternative to shelf-stable prepackaged meals delivered to your doorstep, your local grocery store offers prepared frozen diet meals. If a prepackaged meal by Lean Cuisine (owned by Nestle), Healthy Choice (ConAgra Foods), or Smart Ones (WW) fills you up, you probably weren't that hungry to begin with. Calories in the 170–

340 range are common. And like their shelf-stable counterparts, frozen diet meals contain high levels of preservatives and sodium and they rarely provide enough fruits or vegetables to meet nutritional standards.

Industry Lawsuits Abound

Any time there's big money to be had, profit-driven companies will skirt ethical, legal, and moral lines to gain a competitive advantage. Many lawsuits have been filed against manufacturers of weight loss products for making false or misleading claims, among other misdeeds.

Over a 10-year span (2004–2014), the FTC initiated legal action 82 times against weight loss programs and manufacturers of weight loss products for making false or deceptive claims. The agency collected more than $100M in consumer restitution.[21] The FDA also moved to halt the production and distribution of harmful substances.

Muscletech Research and Development had to cease production of its diet pill Hydroxycut when the FDA banned the use of the stimulant ephedra, which was one of its main ingredients. Ephedra's side effects include heart palpitations, elevated blood pressure, nausea, and vomiting. Among the 800 or so dangerous outcomes from the use of this drug are heart attacks, strokes, seizures, and sudden death.[22] Hydroxycut was later reformulated to rely on high

---

[21] "Fighting on three fronts: FTC weighs in on weight loss ads," FTC.gov (Jun 16, 2014) https://www.ftc.gov/news-events/blogs/business-blog/2014/06/fighting-three-fronts-ftc-weighs-weight-loss-ads

[22] "The dangers of the herb ephedra," Harvard Health Publishing (Jan 20, 2017)

caffeine content, after which many consumers began complaining about elevated heart rate, elevated blood pressure, and loss of sleep, in addition to kidney, cardiovascular, and liver problems.[23]

In 2018, weight loss supplement marketer **Roca Labs** was sued by the FTC for threatening to sue consumers who posted negative reviews about its products online or file complaints with the Better Business Bureau. The FTC also alleged that the company made "false or unsubstantiated weight loss claims and failed to disclose [its] financial ties" to a site where consumers posted positive reviews.[24]

In 2014, the marketer of **Sensa** was fined $26.5M because, as the FTC claimed, the company "deceived consumers with unfounded weight loss claims and misleading endorsements" when it stated that sprinkling the product on food would aid weight loss. Sensa paid the fine but admitted no wrongful conduct.

Around the same time as Sensa's fairy dust lawsuit, several other companies were sued: **HCG Diet Direct**, which marketed an unproven human hormone that was supposed to aid in weight loss; **L'Occitane**, which touted the slimming effect of its skin cream without supporting evidence; and **LeanSpa, LLC,** an operation that (it's alleged) deceptively promoted acai berry and "colon cleanse" weight loss supplements through fake news websites.[25]

---

https://www.health.harvard.edu/staying-healthy/the-dangers-of-the-herb-ephedra
[23] "The Hydroxycut Lawsuit," Impact Law (May 25, 2021) https://www.impactlaw.com/dangerous-drugs/diet-drugs/hydroxycut
[24] "Court Rules in FTC's Favor in Case against Weight-loss Supplement Marketer Roca Labs," FTC.gov (May 25, 2021) https://www.ftc.gov/news-events/press-releases/2018/09/court-rules-ftcs-favor-case-against-weight-loss-supplement
[25] "Sensa and Three Other Marketers of Fad Weight-Loss Products Settle FTC Charges in Crackdown on Deceptive Advertising," FTC.gov (Jan 7, 2014) https://www.ftc.gov/news-events/press-releases/2014/01/sensa-three-other-

Rivalry among competitors has even led to the diet industry suing itself. In 2010, **Weight Watchers** sued **Jenny Craig**, alleging misleading advertising. Admitting no wrongdoing, Jenny Craig agreed to stop running ads that claimed that its weight loss results were twice as effective as its rival's.

I would love to see a class action lawsuit filed on behalf of all the people who've been duped by the empty promises of prepackaged diet foods, meal replacements, programs, and products.

Supplements

Consumers are warned to beware of supplements making weight loss claims.

OxyElite Pro, marketed as a weight loss and muscle-building supplement, was linked to dozens of cases of hepatitis, liver failure requiring liver transplants, and one death.[26]

Fruta Planta Life (Garcinia Cambogia Premium) was found to contain the hidden drug sibutramine, which has been found to significantly increase blood pressure and/or heart rate, as well as potentially interfere with other medications.[27]

Lipozene, a joint venture product between **Obesity Research Institute** and **Continuity Products**, was manufactured and promoted as a supplement claiming to help consumers lose pounds

---

marketers-fad-weight-loss-products-settle-ftc

[26] "LiverTox: Clinical and Research Information on Drug-Induced Liver Injury," National Center for Biotechnology Information (May 20, 2016) https://www.ncbi.nlm.nih.gov/books/NBK548935/

[27] "Public Notification: Fruta Planta contains hidden drug ingredient," FDA.gov (Dec 17, 2020) https://www.fda.gov/drugs/medication-health-fraud/public-notification-fruta-planta-contains-hidden-drug-ingredient

effortlessly. The manufacturers settled a five-year class action lawsuit in 2020 for $4.6M for allegedly making false and misleading claims. The manufacturers admitted no wrongdoing for claiming their product was a "weight loss breakthrough" that would "get rid of pounds of body fat."[28]

The diet supplement problem isn't likely to disappear soon because supplements are much less strictly regulated than many foods and drugs. Indeed, most of the FDA regulations targeting supplements happen only when the FDA hears complaints from consumers after they're already on the market, so it can take months for dangerous items to be removed from the shelves.

Tired of going to court, and as a warning to consumers, the FTC published "The Truth Behind Weight Loss Ads," which did not mince any words. Following are excerpts from that article.

---

[28] "Lipozene Class Action Lawsuit Filed in California," The Senators Firm (Feb 1, 2010) https://www.thesenatorsfirm.com/Law-Blog/2010/February/Lipozene-Class-Action-Lawsuit-Filed-in-Californi.aspx

FTC: The Truth Behind Weight Loss Ads

Dishonest advertisers will say just about anything to get you to buy their weight loss products.

Here are some of the (false) promises from weight loss ads:
- Lose weight without dieting or exercising. (You won't.)
- You don't have to watch what you eat to lose weight. (You do.)
- If you use this product, you'll lose weight permanently. (Wrong.)
- To lose weight, all you have to do is take this pill. (Not true.)
- You can lose 30 pounds in 30 days. (Nope.)
- This product works for everyone. (It doesn't.)
- Lose weight with this patch or cream. (You can't.)

Here's the truth:
- Any promise of miraculous weight loss is simply untrue.
- No product will let you eat all the food you want and still lose weight.
- Permanent weight loss requires permanent lifestyle changes, so don't trust any product that promises once-and-for-all results.
- Products promising lightning-fast weight loss are always a scam. Worse, they can ruin your health.
- Even if a product could help some people lose weight in

some situations, there's no one-size-fits-all product guaranteed to work for everyone. Everyone's habits and health concerns are unique.
- Nothing you can wear or apply to your skin will cause you to lose weight. Period.[29]

The Biggest Losers

So, if weight loss products, pills, supplements, creams, potions, and meal replacements don't work, we should just reduce our calories and work out ridiculously hard. That must be the solution. Right? Nowhere has this "solution" been more rigorously tested than on the TV show *The Biggest Loser*.

On *The Biggest Loser*, contestants who have excess pounds in the triple digits experience dramatic weight loss over a 30-week period. Eureka! It can be done! It just requires an around-the-clock team of trainers and nutritionists, the risk of worldwide embarrassment, and a monetary carrot at the end of the treadmill. Not to mention the contestants' dedication, persistence, sacrifice, and grueling hard work.

Not only is the *Biggest Loser* not doable for most of us, the "final" results shared on the show are anything but. At a scheduled six-year checkup of 14 of the show's contestants, the National Institute of Health (NIH) found that, although the group members' starting weight had gone from an average of 328 pounds, to a low weight of 200 as the contest wrapped up, they had each regained most of that

---

[29] "The Truth Behind Weight Loss Ads," Consumer.FTC.gov (May 25, 2021) https://www.consumer.ftc.gov/articles/truth-behind-weight-loss-ads

weight, ending up at an average of 290 pounds.[30] Their body fat percentage, which had dropped from 49% to 28% on average during the contest, now averaged 45%. Only one of the 14 contestants kept most of the weight off, and four were heavier than before the competition began.

An even sadder story was told by the contestants' metabolism. While the group averaged a burn rate of 2,667 calories per day at the start of the competition, burn rate had dropped to 2,000 calories per day at the competition's end, and at the NIH checkup, it had slid further to 1,900 calories on average. This means they were required to eat less than they could before their weight loss to avoid gaining weight.

This is also true for most dieters who successfully lose weight. And beyond the deprivation and the wasted time, money, and effort, weight loss failures also take a mental and psychological toll on us. A study published in the journal *Psychosomatic Medicine* found that dieting doesn't work, with most dieters gaining back all the weight they lose. Worse, they then suffered psychological issues, such as stress, anxiety, lowered self-esteem, depression, and irritability.

Damned straight, we're irritable.

In the US, it's estimated that 45 million people go on a diet each year. Most will fail to lose any significant amount of weight. For

---

[30] Kathryn Doyle, "6 Years After The Biggest Loser, Metabolism Is Slower and Weight is Back Up," *Scientific American* (May 10, 2016)
https://www.scientificamerican.com/article/6-years-after-the-biggest-loser-metabolism-is-slower-and-weight-is-back-up/

those who do lose weight, 80% will regain it within 12 months. This appalling failure rate creates a perpetual, reliable, and surprisingly loyal market for the weight loss industry.

Aren't we being just a little naïve? What other industry has an 80% failure rate and yet continues to attract the same customers year after year? The definition of insanity is doing the same thing over and over and expecting to fit into a size 4.

The gain/lose cycle is a hamster wheel of profits perpetuated by huge advertising budgets. On one hand, we have the media bombarding us with messages that slender is beautiful, skinny is sexy, and svelte signifies success. This creates the market for diet products and services.

On the other hand, we're inundated with advertisements for fast food, sugary foods, deep-fried foods, carb-loaded foods, and highly processed, prepackaged, low-nutrition food-like substances. And after we've scarfed down mocha Frappuccinos and Godiva chocolates and artisan garlic loaves like dutiful consumers, we're told we're too fat and we'd better lose weight, so here's a new plan, cutting-edge program, breakthrough supplement, no-fail pill, ultimate workout DVD, or miracle cream that's sure to make us look like Gwyneth Paltrow within six weeks for only four easy payments of $49.95. *Insert, slide, or wave your credit card here. Thank you for your business. Have a nice day!*

And when our efforts fail (again), the fashion industry is there to have us SPANXed. Suck it in, tuck it in, girls. That discomfort you're feeling is the price you pay for your overindulgence. After all, it's the science, stupid. All you have to do is burn more calories than you take in, and you'll lose weight. Everybody knows that! So, you must not be trying, tracking, or treadmilling hard enough. You must be cheating. You must be *lazy*.

At some point, we either redouble our efforts (and fail twice as fast) or throw in our sweat-drenched workout towel, probably at the mirror, and preferably with a rock in it. We give up, we give in, and we decide we're going to accept being overweight and the accompanying health risks.

Or we go for the drastic solution—weight loss surgery.

Weight Loss Surgery

Bariatric surgery is the collective name for the most common weight loss surgeries, which include Roux-en-Y, mini-gastric bypass, lap banding, and sleeve. The Mayo Clinic posts this definition of bariatric surgery on its site:

> "Bariatric surgery is done when diet and exercise haven't worked or when you have serious health problems because of your weight. Some procedures limit how much you can eat. Other procedures work by reducing the body's ability to absorb nutrients. Some procedures do both.
>
> "While bariatric surgery can offer many benefits, all forms of weight-loss surgery are major procedures that can pose serious risks and side effects. Also, you must make permanent healthy changes to your diet and get regular exercise to help ensure the long-term success of bariatric surgery."

A couple of phrases jump out: "... reducing the body's ability to absorb nutrients" and "... major procedures that can pose serious risks and side effects." But the statement that slays is the last bit: "You must make permanent healthy changes to your diet and get regular exercise to help ensure the long-term success of bariatric surgery."[31]

So, we undergo an expensive and invasive medical procedure that carries serious health risks and side effects, and at the end of the rainbow, we're right back at square one and are advised to change our diet and get regular exercise to maintain this "success"? Pass the ketchup, please. My fries are getting lonely.

Let's review what each of these procedures entails.

Roux-en-Y

Roux-en-Y is better known as a gastric bypass. It's one of the more commonly performed procedures (mainly because some insurers will cover it under specific conditions), and it can be done either laparoscopically (through small cuts in your abdomen) or robotically (using computer-assisted surgery).[32] With a gastric bypass, the surgeon separates the upper portion of your stomach from the lower portion. Your upper portion now becomes a pouch which is

---

[31] "Bariatric Surgery," Mayo Clinic (May 25, 2021) https://www.mayoclinic.org/tests-procedures/bariatric-surgery/about/pac-20394258

[32] "Roux-en-Y Gastric Bypass (RYGB)," University of Illinois Hospital (May 25, 2021) https://hospital.uillinois.edu/primary-and-specialty-care/surgical-services/bariatric-surgery-program/our-services/roux-en-y-gastric-bypass-rygb

then connected to a branch of your small intestine. This new pouch limits the amount of food you can eat, making you feel full after eating only a small amount. Once this pouch is created, the surgeon then reroutes your digestive system to bypass the rest of your stomach and part of your small intestine. This allows you to absorb fewer calories and nutrients from the food you eat, which is defined as *malabsorption*. Cost of a gastric bypass: $25,000.

Mini-gastric bypass

The **mini-gastric bypass** is a slightly quicker procedure. Here's one insurance advisor's definition of mini-gastric bypass surgery:

1. The stomach is divided with a laparoscopic stapler. Most of the stomach is no longer attached to the esophagus and will no longer receive food. Your new stomach is much smaller and shaped like a small tube.
2. Between 2 to 7 feet of intestines are bypassed. The surgeon will attach the remainder of the intestines to the new stomach.
3. Food now flows into your small tube-like stomach and then bypasses between 2 to 7 feet of intestines where it resumes the normal digestive process in ... the remaining intestine. [33]

---

[33] OC Staff, "Mini-Gastric Bypass – The Good, Bad, And Ugly," Obesity Coverage (June 4, 2020) https://www.obesitycoverage.com/mini-gastric-bypass-the-good-bad-and-ugly/

The mini-gastric bypass is believed to potentially carry less risk than the traditional bypass simply because it reroutes less of your intestine, but it does carry one additional risk as compared to its big brother counterpart: biliary (bile) reflux. Because the pouch is smaller and the rest of your stomach is still attached to your intestines, it's possible for gastric juices to travel down your intestines and into the new pouch. Cost of a mini-gastric bypass: $16,000–$20,000.

Lap band surgery

Laparoscopic adjustable gastric banding (LAGB, or lap band surgery) is a surgical procedure that involves placing an adjustable "belt" around the upper portion of your stomach. The belt can be tightened by adding saline to fill it (like blowing air into a child's swimming pool floatie). The belt is connected to a port that is placed under the skin of your stomach. This port is used to add or remove saline from the belt. Lap band surgery limits the size of your stomach and the amount of food it can hold, and it slows the passage of food to your intestines. Cost of lap band surgery: $15,000. Side effects include "… nausea, vomiting, ulceration at the band site, esophageal reflux (indigestion), weight regain, and dehydration … Constipation is commonly encountered."[34]

---

[34] "Lap Band Surgery Side Effects," MedicineNet (Sept 16, 2020) https://www.medicinenet.com/lap_band_surgery_gastric_banding/article.htm

Gastric sleeve surgery

Gastric sleeve surgery is usually performed laparoscopically. The surgeon removes 75-80% of your stomach, leaving a small tube-shaped "sleeve" that can hold much less food. Unlike gastric bypass surgeries, this surgery can't be reversed because most of your stomach is gone. As with a gastric bypass, patients are at risk for long-term nutrient deficiencies. And, as you may recall from your biology class, nutrients are essential to a healthy functioning body.

> Shrinking someone's stomach to the size of a walnut with surgery is one way to battle obesity and diabetes … but it doesn't address the underlying causes.
>
> **Mark Hyman, MD**

One reason sleeve surgery is effective for weight loss is that by removing most of the stomach, the body's level of ghrelin, a hormone commonly called the "hunger hormone," is reduced. And because ghrelin also plays a role in blood sugar metabolism, those with type 2 diabetes often have an immediate decrease in their need for diabetes medications after the procedure. We'll discuss the hunger-signaling of ghrelin later, but it has a much larger role to play in our bodies than this.

If you're thinking that living without most of your stomach and nutrient deficiency is a small price to pay to lose that muffin top, consider that risks include indigestion, sagging skin, gallstones, stomach ulcers, nausea, addiction transfer, and gastroesophageal reflux disease (GERD). GERD occurs when stomach acid frequently flows back into the esophagus, which is the tube that connects your mouth and your stomach. This backwash can irritate the lining of your esophagus, not to mention take all the joy out of kissing. Wondering about addiction transfer? It can happen with any of the bariatric surgeries. Here's a quick definition of addiction transfer from the Obesity Action Coalition:

> "Addiction transfer, or cross addiction, after bariatric surgery occurs when individuals trade compulsive eating for other compulsive behaviors. There is also strong evidence of a biological reason for cross addiction.
>
> "Studies show various forms of transfer addiction in up to 30 percent of patients who have had bariatric surgery. For these patients, food is no longer being a source of comfort, distraction, reward, or escape. Other behaviors or substances now substitute for eating, and can become problematic." [35]

In addition to the risks of indigestion, sagging skin, gallstones, stomach ulcers, nausea, addiction transfer, and GERD, over time, a gastric sleeve stretches. As it stretches, it's able to take in larger and larger amounts of food, allowing larger meals to be consumed, which can lead to weight regain. Cost of gastric sleeve surgery: about $15,000.

---

[35] "Transfer Addiction Following Bariatric Surgery," Obesity Action Coalition (April 19, 2016) https://www.obesityaction.org/community/news/bariatric-surgery/transfer-addiction-following-bariatric-surgery/

Surgery by the numbers

In 2019, 278,000 people had some form of bariatric surgery in the US. This was an increase of 50,000 patients from 2017 numbers. Before the pandemic, the number of bariatric surgeries had been projected 2020 numbers to reach 297,000.

In extreme cases, bariatric surgery is a life-saving procedure. But it's a very drastic step to take, carrying lifelong consequences and serious health risks. It's reasonable that some would take this step when "all else" has failed, and many bariatric surgery patients *have* tried dieting and exercise and failed. But in most cases, they failed because weight loss due to caloric restriction *sets us up for failure*; it reduces our metabolism because *it must*. Our bodies aren't stupid, and nature doesn't make mistakes.

When I was I grad school, we read a short story about a king and a hawk by James Baldwin. In the story, the king dips his cup into a stream and tries to take a drink of water, but his pet hawk swoops down and knocks the cup from his hand. Twice the hawk does this, as the king's anger mounts. On the third pass, the king draws his sword and kills the hawk. Only after this fit of rage does he see the huge poisonous snake lying dead in the water. The hawk had been trying to save him.

When our bodies receive fewer calories, they adjust and begin burning fewer calories. And this is a very good thing! Our bodies want us to keep living. To ensure that, they slow our burn rate to protect us. And yet, we scream at our bathroom scales and curse our own dear bodies for this natural process of self-protection. We may not kill the hawk, but we often hate it.

Instead of fighting or rallying against our bodies for doing what they're supposed to do to ensure our survival, wouldn't it be great if we could somehow learn how to communicate *with* our bodies to get them to do what we want them to do: lose weight, retain muscle, and lose fat without sacrificing our metabolism?

Exercise Isn't the Answer

Exercise is part of a healthy lifestyle; it's good for our cardiovascular health, our bone strength, our overall conditioning, and our mental wellbeing. But it isn't the answer to weight loss.

In an article on Vox.com[36] titled "The science is in: Exercise won't help you lose much weight," the author reported on 60 exercise and weight loss studies. These studies found basic metabolic rate and food digestion account for 60-90% of our energy expenditure, leaving a mere 10-30% for physical activity. This 10-30% includes all movement we do throughout the day, whether it's labeled exercise or not. The author concluded, "... if one is overweight or obese, and presumably trying to lose dozens of pounds, it would take an incredible amount of time, will, and effort to make a real impact through exercise alone."

---

[36] Julia Belluz and Christophe Haubursin, "The science is in: exercise won't help you lose much weight," Vox.com (Jan 2, 2019) https://www.vox.com/2018/1/3/16845438/exercise-weight-loss-myth-burn-calories

Many studies (and perhaps your own study of one) also find that people tend to increase their food intake after exercise and, as unfair as it seems, a single slice of pizza can undo an hour's workout.

That's all the bad news. You may have suspected much of that based on your own experience.

Now the Good News

The good news is, it is possible to lose weight and fat permanently once we understand how our bodies work. We can:

- Drop the weight,
- Drop the fat,
- Retain our muscle, and
- Increase our metabolism

And that's not even the best part. The same solution for effective, life-affirming weight loss provides much bigger results.

With this type of slim fast solution (small *s*, small *f*), we can work with our bodies to help reverse or prevent type 2 diabetes and prediabetes, perform cellular repair, prevent age-related diseases such as Alzheimer's, and reduce our risk for cancer, stroke, and mental decline.

Who knew? Fung knew.

CHAPTER 3

You've Got A Friend in Fung

ENTER DR. JASON FUNG. No one has done more to dispel the myth that a calorie-restricted diet + exercise = weight loss than Dr. Fung.

Dr. Fung is a Canadian nephrologist, a specialist who works with kidney patients. In his practice, he has treated thousands of type 2 diabetes patients who were either on dialysis or heading there. He's shared what he's learned about intermittent fasting (IF) through several best-selling health books including *The Obesity Code*, *The Diabetes Code*, *The Cancer Code*, and *The Complete Guide to Fasting*. I recommend you read one or more of these books, or at least visit his website, thefastingmethod.com. Dr. Fung is co-founder of the Intensive Dietary Management Program, which he uses at his clinic in Toronto to treat patients suffering from type 2 diabetes and obesity.

Please go to the source by checking out his books, YouTube videos, and online articles for the science behind what I'm about to share. I'm a layperson, not a doctor or a scientist. My goal in this chapter is to explain what I've learned about intermittent fasting in easily digestible (no pun intended) terms so that when you hear it from Dr. Fung, more of what he says will sink in. However, you'll find that he does a great job of simplifying it, too.

Weight gain can cause a Humvee's worth of bodily ailments. When it leads to type 2 diabetes, it can kill you slowly, rotting your body parts, blinding you ... it's a *Little Shop of Horrors*, with the disease as the carnivorous plant.

Dr. Fung's advancements in treating weight gain and obesity are a direct outcome of his work with type 2 diabetes patients. So, let's start there and work our way back to solving the weight puzzle once and for all. For some readers, this may seem like a side issue, but I promise I'll make the connection. And for those who have been diagnosed with type 2 diabetes or prediabetes (as I was), this will have special relevance.

Both type 1 and type 2 diabetes are collectively called diabetes mellitus, but they are very different diseases. Type 2 symptoms can include the following:

- Increased thirst
- Frequent urination
- Increased hunger
- Unintended weight loss

- Fatigue
- Blurred vision
- Slow-healing sores
- Frequent infections
- Numbness or tingling in the hands or feet
- Areas of darkened skin, usually in the armpits and neck
- Sexual dysfunction
- Diabetic coma
- Heart disease
- Stroke
- Gum disease
- Kidney disease
- Diabetic neuropathy and subsequent amputation
- Blindness
- Death

Until recently, type 2 diabetes was known as *adult-onset diabetes* because it was seen almost exclusively in adults, whereas type 1 was almost exclusively diagnosed in children. According to the Mayo Clinic, however, an increase in obesity in children has led to an increase in type 2 diabetes in them as well.[37]

---

[37] "Type 2 Diabetes," Mayo Clinic (May 25, 2021) https://www.mayoclinic.org/diseases-conditions/type-2-diabetes/symptoms-causes/syc-20351193

Customary Treatment for Type 2 Diabetes

Type 2 diabetes occurs when the body produces so much insulin that its receptors become resistant to it (insulin resistance) and fail to use it properly. We'll get to exactly *why* the body produces too much insulin in a moment. The medical solution for an over-abundance of insulin when treating type 2 diabetes? More insulin. Does this make any sense?

Let's say you're vacationing at a cabin in the woods, and you need to go to the woodpile and carry firewood to heat the cabin. You're outside picking up more firewood than you can possibly carry, and, as you walk toward the cabin, some pieces of firewood begin to drop from your arms. So, your helpful cabin mate keeps stacking more and more wood on top, and it keeps falling off, and your mate keeps stacking more, and the cycle continues until your cabin mate gets tired of this game and stalks off.

The problem you have in this scenario is that you're carrying too much firewood, and you can't solve that problem by carrying more firewood. So, let's get back to our question: Why do type 2 diabetes patients produce too much insulin? And, while we're at it, what is insulin, and what does it do?

Food consists of *carbohydrates, proteins*, and *fats*. Carbohydrates are absorbed by our bodies and turned into glucose; this raises blood sugar levels. The pancreas produces insulin to manage the glucose. Insulin enables glucose to enter our cells, which then convert it into glycogen or fat and use it as energy. In its transportation role, insulin controls how much glucose (blood sugar) is in our bloodstream at any given moment by shuttling it out of our bloodstream and into our cells. Insulin helps store glucose in our liver, fat, and muscles. The higher our glucose level, the more insulin our pancreas must produce to manage it.

When a lot of blood sugar (glucose) enters our bloodstream, our helpful pancreas pumps out more insulin to make sure that the glucose gets into our cells. Like your helpful cabin mate, your insulin delivers more and more blood sugar to the cell walls. But just as your arms can only carry so much firewood, your cells can only hold so much glycogen, and after a while they stop responding to insulin's attempts to shove more glucose in. When cells stop responding to insulin, they've become insulin resistant. The pancreas notices that there's still plenty of glucose in the bloodstream, so it keeps pumping out more insulin to deal with it. But like your helpful cabin mate, the pancreas will eventually tire of this game, too.

Here's another analogy: a classic episode from the comedy show, *I Love Lucy*. In this episode, Lucy and Ethel had taken jobs at a chocolate factory and were tasked with wrapping chocolates in paper as the chocolates were being spit out by a conveyor belt. At first, they found the task easy, but when the conveyor belt sped up, they couldn't cope. Panicked, they began to stuff the chocolate anywhere: into their apron pockets, into their mouths, down their shirts, but it was a losing battle. The conveyor belt won. When glucose is coming at us too fast, our body produces more insulin to try to keep up. But like Lucy and Ethel, there's only so much our body can do, and eventually, our cells can't fit any more glucose in, so they ignore the insulin.

In the beginning, when our body ignores insulin, the pancreas thinks we just need more insulin, and the conveyor belt keeps coming. At first, this is somewhat effective, with the sheer quantity of insulin delivered acting as a sort of battering ram.

The ability of the pancreas to ramp up insulin production is why people with insulin resistance won't show any symptoms at first. If you've been diagnosed with prediabetes, it means your blood glucose levels are outside of the normal range but aren't yet high enough for you to be classified as diabetic. This elevated glucose level happens because your pancreas slows down production of insulin or because your body isn't using insulin as well as it should. When glucose can't enter the cells, a higher level of sugar builds up in the blood, which is called *hyperglycemia*. And when the body is unable to use the glucose for energy, this leads to the symptoms of type 2 diabetes. Without effective intervention, the cells become starved for nutrients and begin cellular death, leading to neuropathy and, often foot ulcers. Every year, surgeons

> Insulin resistance can happen due to a combination of genetics and lifestyle leading to an inflammatory process in the body. There are many biological stress factors that can set insulin resistance in motion, including excess nutrition."
>
> **Obesity Medicine**

perform lower-limb amputations due to diabetes on about 73,000 patients. Most of these amputations are performed to treat non-healing diabetic foot ulcers.[38]

The traditional treatment for insulin deficiency has been to target blood sugar levels—the symptom of the disease, not the disease itself. So, even when blood sugar levels are brought under control by the application of more insulin, the disease itself doesn't get better and frequently gets worse. Because the disease worsens in most type 2 diabetes patients who are treated by applying more insulin, type 2 diabetes has been thought to be a chronic, progressive, and irreversible disease.

> [Insulin] is the wrong treatment. And if you give the wrong treatment, guess what? Everybody dies.
>
> **Dr. Jason Fung**

Dr. Fung discovered that, while most of his patients' symptoms worsened, those who eliminated sugar and most carbs both lost weight and saw a reduction in their type 2 diabetes symptoms. In many cases, they were able to reverse their symptoms and get off their diabetes medication entirely. This and their accompanying weight loss were contrary to the prevailing medical paradigm, which said that it was fat, not carbs, that caused weight gain. And it said that type 2 diabetes was chronic and irreversible.

---

[38] "The Unfortunate and Avoidable Truth About Foot Amputation Due to Diabetes," Azura Vascular Care (Feb 16, 2017) https://www.azuravascularcare.com/infopad/foot-amputation-due-to-diabetes/

Around this same time, some notable medical journals, including *The New England Journal of Medicine*, published studies on how high-carb, low-fat diets weren't effective for weight loss, and in fact, better results were seen with low-carb, high-fat diets—not just for weight loss but for improvements across all important risk factors for cardiovascular disease, including cholesterol, blood sugar level, and blood pressure. These reports, plus the results he was seeing in his own clinic, caused Dr. Fung to investigate further.

By now, we all know (even if only based on our own empirical evidence of one) that "calories in, calories out" diets don't work, either. Let's look at why.

Three Key Hormones

To understand why the calories in, calories out model is fatally flawed, we need to understand the function of three primary hormones: *insulin*, *ghrelin*, which, as we mentioned, puts the *grr* in hunger, and *leptin*.

Think of leptin as ghrelin's opposite. Ghrelin says, "You're hungry. Eat something already!" The hormone leptin travels from your fat cells to your brain and says, "You've had enough. Stop eating!" So, if leptin is produced by fat cells, shouldn't it be doing its messenger job a whole lot better, notifying us that we've had enough and can stop eating? When leptin isn't doing its job, it's because of an overabundance of ... insulin. Insulin prevents it from delivering that message.

By now, insulin is starting to sound like the dastardly villain in those old cartoons, right? Insulin can have life-saving benefits for those with type 1 diabetes, but for the rest of us, too much of it has us tied to the railroad tracks, and the train is coming.

Insulin blocks leptin, so we don't get the message that we've eaten enough. At the same time, insulin has been shown to *increase* the circulation of *ghrelin*, the hunger hormone. *Choo choo.*

When type 2 diabetes patients are given insulin, their blood sugar (glucose) levels go down, but where does the glucose go? It's no longer in the bloodstream because insulin (and its new insulin reinforcements) has rammed it into fat for storage. An abundance of insulin makes us fat. The more insulin we have, the more fat we store.

You might be thinking, "Wait a minute ... No one's pumping ME full of insulin, and I've got plenty of fat I'd like to lose." Actually, someone *is* pumping you full of insulin, and I'm sorry to report that this person is you. The good news is, if you're doing it, you have the power to stop doing it. And it won't require a pill, a program, or a pedometer. In fact, it won't cost you a cent.

What Dr. Fung Discovered

After further research, Dr. Fung dramatically changed how he treated his type 2 diabetes patients—many of whom also struggled with obesity. The treatment he discovered worked to solve *both* conditions. The key wasn't removing glucose from the bloodstream by adding more insulin. The key was removing glucose from the bloodstream and glycogen from the body—which meant getting it out of our fat stores. This was no easy feat because our bodies prefer glycogen as a food source. Our bodies will always go for glycogen first, and unless and until it's depleted, they will continue to prefer glycogen, meaning our fat stays right where it is. The only way to get at fat stores is to deplete glycogen completely so our bodies have no choice but to start burning fat. The two ways to do that are:

- Fasting
- Following a very low-carbohydrate, high-fat diet (such as the ketogenic diet)

Why Fasting Works

When we fast, our insulin levels drop, which tells our body to start burning stored energy. Because glycogen is the most easily accessed energy source, it gets burned first. Our liver stores enough glycogen to provide energy for 24–36 hours. Once that's depleted, our body turns to our stored fat for energy. Getting at stored fat is impossible without glycogen depletion. Dr. Fung uses a helpful analogy to explain this: the refrigerator and the basement freezer.

Think of your glycogen as the food in your refrigerator. It's where you'll go first to make a meal. If you keep grocery shopping (filling your body with glycogen), your refrigerator will always have a ready supply, and there will be no need to tap into your basement freezer. You simply can't access it until that refrigerator is depleted.

Our bodies are always either storing or burning food energy. If we're constantly in the storing and burning mode, every time we eat a little more than we burn, we're going to gain weight. If we want to shed pounds and reduce fat, we must reduce the amount of storing we do, and the simplest way to do that is to fast.

Before you say, "I could never fast!" know this: *You already fast every single day when you're sleeping.* When you wake, you "break" your "fast." Hence, the name for what's erroneously called the most important meal of the day, breakfast. More on that later.

Delaying your first meal of the day simply extends your usual nightly fast. The longer you delay, the more your body will rely on stored fat for energy once your glycogen levels are depleted. The more you can reduce your insulin, the more fat you will lose.

Fasting isn't "fun," per se. But I can attest to this: Sometimes you do enjoy it. And it gets easier the more you do it because your body becomes "fat adapted," allowing you to switch from burning glycogen to burning fat more easily, particularly if you eat mostly healthy food (lower carb, higher fat) overall. And here's the great news: When your body is fat adapted, you can often tap into that basement freezer even when there's food left in the fridge.

Intermittent Fasting Defined

Intermittent fasting isn't "not eating"—it's scheduling *when* you eat. For that reason, it's also known as time-restricted eating. Between your scheduled eating times, you avoid all food except no-calorie beverages that don't contain artificial sweeteners. Besides water, this may include black coffee, tea, and mineral water. While not strictly water fasts, coffee, tea, etc., contain no (or very few) calories and won't "break" your fast. However, shun artificial sweeteners for all kinds of health reasons.

If you can avoid eating for one hour, you've basically done intermittent fasting. Will one hour without food give you the results you want? Unlikely. Finding your own comfort level with intermittent fasting—and knowing the body benefits you'll reap—is the subject of the next chapter. Meet you there!

More to Know

"Your body is like a sugar bowl. It can hold a certain amount of sugar. But if you keep filling it with sugar, it spills out into the blood. Adding insulin doesn't get rid of the sugar in the blood; it crams it back into the body; next time you eat, the sugar bowl is still full [cycle repeats]—you haven't fixed the problem—so you keep having to take more insulin. After 10–20 years, your whole body starts to rot: eyes go, gangrene, foot ulcers, kidneys start to go."

— **Dr. Jason Fung**, *A New Paradigm of Insulin Resistance* (YouTube)

Fung on Type 2 Diabetes

"We can actually completely cure the whole damned disease ... and if you don't have [type 2] diabetes, you don't have neuropathy, foot ulcers, diabetic retinopathy, stroke, cancers, MI [myocardial infarction] ... No drugs, no surgery, no cost."

—**Dr. Jason Fung**, *Beginner's Guide to Intermittent Fasting* (YouTube)

Glucose vs. Glycogen: What's the Difference?

Glucose (blood sugar) is a monosaccharide. Insulin helps convert glucose into glycogen (a polysaccharide) and fat. In fat cells, insulin helps promote the uptake of glucose and its conversion into fat. In the liver, insulin converts glucose into glycogen and into fat. The liver is limited in the amount of glycogen that it can store, so the muscles help. In muscle cells, insulin promotes glucose as fuel and stores it a glycogen. Approximately one-third of glucose that travels through the liver is converted to fatty acids and stored as adipose (fat tissue).

Insulin's job is to facilitate glucose entry into cells for energy conversion. When cells get full or have all they can handle, additional glucose is rushed to fat cells to be stored as triglycerides. So, when insulin is high, the body is UNABLE to burn fat.

Sugar: Our Favorite Poison

The **World Health Organization** recommends limiting sugar to no more than **six teaspoons per day**. Americans are eating on average 130 pounds a year, which equals **38.73 teaspoons per day**. This includes consumption of high fructose corn syrup (HFCS).

Our overconsumption of sugar, a toxin, has been called a "public health crisis" by Dr. Robert Lustig, pediatric endocrinologist at the

University of California. He says we should treat sugar similarly to how we treat tobacco and alcohol: "... sugar belongs in the same wastebasket."

CHAPTER 4

IF, OMAD, ADF, WTF?

ONE SIGNIFICANT BENEFIT of IF (intermittent fasting) is that you can fit it around your life, rather than trying to fit your life around a rigid diet. You can eat cake! Marie Antoinette would approve![39] You can have wine. I approve!

Overall good health comes from making predominantly good choices about what you put into your body. But you can still enjoy happy hours and pizza and French fries and chocolate. Just enjoy these in moderation and don't make them the staples of your diet. And in between eating mostly healthy foods with occasional treats, you fast on a schedule that works for you.

---

[39] Many scholars doubt she said this. (Maybe it was Sara Lee.)

The Difference Between Fasting and Starvation

You're not going to starve when you fast. Starving is *involuntary* food abstinence. If a starving person were presented with a nice plate of food, even a somewhat *unappetizing* plate of food, she would eat! Fasting is *voluntary* food abstinence. You're in complete control of when you next eat, which in fasting vernacular is the beginning of your "feeding window." As we've covered, fasting can be as simple as delaying your first meal after you wake up. Let's look at some common schedules for fasting.

The 16:8 Method

I think of the 16:8 method as the gateway fast. With 16:8, you fast for 16 hours and eat for eight. Your first 16 hours include the eight hours when you're sleeping and the several hours after dinner before you go to bed, so it's comfortable for most people. For instance, you could stop eating at 7 p.m. and decide not to eat again until 16 hours later, which would be 11 a.m. the next day.

That doesn't sound so bad, does it? Are you going to want a snack late at night? Probably. Are you going to get hungry before 11 a.m.? Probably. Your body may be used to snacking at night and eating breakfast soon after you wake up, and while fasting, you're not snacking and you're delaying breakfast until "brunch." But here's the thing: Hunger comes in waves. A wave of hunger is our stomach signaling us that we didn't eat when it expected to receive food, and that signal is a gentle reminder. If we ignore it, it will go away. You've probably experienced this before: You've been hungry, but got busy, and the hunger went away. With fasting, you consciously ignore the hunger. And it does go away. It doesn't hurt to keep yourself busy or distracted by other things.

The 20:4 Method

As you can probably guess, the 20:4 method simply extends your fasting period another four hours to 20 hours and compresses your eating into a four-hour window, say from 4 p.m. to 8 p.m. This is similar to the Warrior Diet, which you may have heard of. The idea is that warriors don't have time to eat, and when they do eat, they *really* eat, mostly lots of protein and fats. But you can eat whatever you want in your feeding window; it doesn't have to be the head of a yak.

One Meal a Day (OMAD)

The One Meal a Day method is similar to the 20:4 method, but instead of a four-hour feeding window, you compress your feeding window into a single meal. This can be any meal that works for you, but when I do OMAD, I've found that dinner works best for me because if I eat too early, that leaves a whole stretch of time before bed that I'm not eating. Why do that to myself?

Another benefit to having dinner as your one meal a day is that this tends to be the time when you socialize with family. Will you overeat during that one meal? You may, but you likely won't eat a whole day's worth of calories in one meal. And even if you did, your body has still reaped the many health benefits of fasting, which we'll cover later in this chapter.

The 5/2 Method

Unlike its name suggests, the 5/2 method isn't eating for five hours and fasting for two! With this method, you eat normally five days of the week and fast on any two days that work for you. These can be back-to-back, say Tuesday/Wednesday, or they can be separated by a few days, such as Monday/Thursday. On the two fasting days, you can eat up to 500 calories. Many people love this method. I often do 5/2 myself, but instead of eating those 500 calories, I abstain from all food on my fasting days. This isn't because I have such amazing willpower (quite the opposite)! It's because if I eat something, I get my gastric juices going, and that makes me want to eat more. Just knowing that I'm not eating at all that day and can eat the next day works better for me. But you do you!

Alternate Day Fasting (ADF)

I used ADF to lose significant weight in preparation for my nephew's wedding. I lost 30 pounds and got into a size 2 Calvin Klein dress! It was pretty easy, and I looked forward to my fasting days because I didn't have to think about what I was going to eat. As the name implies, you eat one day and fast the next. On the days I ate, I kept it in the healthy range, plus occasional Mai Tais. I also exercised regularly on both eating and fasting days: walking and a mini-trampoline workout I'll share later.

ADF has a sibling: modified ADF. With modified ADF, you can consume up to 500 calories (make them healthy)! This is similar to the 5/2 method, but you're switching it up so the "2" becomes every other day.

Extended Fasts

I've also done extended day fasts, which have such amazing health benefits it's ridiculous. As mentioned, it sometimes takes 24–36 hours to start getting into your fat stores. Fasts of 48 hours or more can ensure you're emptying out that deep freezer. I've done several three-day fasts and one five-day fast. And to prepare for this book, just so I could report on the process, I decided to do a 14-day fast, which I'll report on later.

Extended day fasts aren't dangerous if you do them right! Drink your water, take a food-based multivitamin, and make sure you're getting your electrolytes (very important, but skip the Gatorade, please!). We'll discuss how to support a longer fast later. There's no real need to be concerned about electrolytes or supplementation on shorter, intermittent fasts.

Dry Fasting and Dirty Fasting

Two other forms of fasting I should mention are dry fasting and dirty fasting. *Dry fasting* means you take in nothing—not even water. Some people swear by the health benefits of dry fasting, but I'm not (yet) a believer. Health experts drill it into our brains how important it is to drink water, and now we're supposed to go without? I've never tried it and have no plans to do so. Many of those who do dry fasting also do skin brushing, which is good for you regardless of whether you're fasting. Skin brushing is a daily body massage with a dry, stiff-bristled brush. It hurts! However, it can help remove dead skin, increase circulation, detoxify, help digestion – and, according to some, even improve the appearance of cellulite. I keep a boar bristle brush in the shower and use it *after* soaping up. It's still moderately painful, but it's bearable.

Dirty fasting is allowing yourself some calories while you fast. Depending on how big of a purist a faster is, this could include a bit of half-and-half in your coffee, a small salad or veggies, or a handful of nuts. I don't do dirty fasting for the same reason I don't eat on my 2 days when I do 5/2. For me, eating leads to more eating. When I fast, I'm all in. I do drink black coffee, which is still a "clean" fast even though it has 2 calories a cup. I burn more than that grinding the beans.

Mix & Match

Fasting is flexible! There's nothing to say that you can't mix and match different fasting plans to suit your lifestyle and goals. I know one woman who dropped 30 pounds in four months by combining ADF with IF (her feeding window was 11 a.m. to 6 p.m. eating whole foods ("nothing in a can or box," she said) and combined that with two 72-hour fasts per month. "Several weeks I didn't feel like doing ADF so I just did IF." Flexibility will keep you from feeling like you "blew it" if you don't stick to your plan, which is demoralizing and can send you off the rails. You are always in control of your plan.

Maintenance

Even if weight loss isn't your goal, I hope by now you see that fasting is great for your overall health. However, if weight loss is a goal, you may be thinking, "But when I stop, won't I gain it all back?" Sure, if you go back to your former eating patterns. But fasting is great for weight maintenance!

Find what works for you. You may start with IF three days a week. If you find the weight creeping back on, extend that to five, or add in one fasting day per week.

Who Shouldn't Fast?

Pregnant and breastfeeding women, those with eating disorders such as anorexia, and those who are already underweight should not fast. Those with type 2 diabetes should only fast under their doctor's care because, as Dr. Fung's practice showed, fasting can reduce (and eventually eliminate) the need for insulin, and your medication may need to be adjusted. And people on other forms of medication that must be taken with food should also consult with their doctor before beginning a fasting program. It's possible your medications can be timed to coincide with your feeding window, so ask.

Busting Myths

Myth: Fasting is starvation
Fasting is *not* starvation. We've already covered that. You can stop any time you want and eat. Fasting has been done for thousands of years as both a spiritual practice and as a matter of practicality when

food was scarce. In modern times, the longest record of a person fasting is 382 days. A Scottish gentleman, Angus Barbieri, fasted from June 1965 to July 1966, subsisting on tea, coffee, soda water (for the electrolytes), and a multivitamin. He occasionally allowed himself small amounts of milk or sugar with his beverages, mostly near the end of his fast, and he was frequently evaluated by a local hospital throughout his fast. He had been obese and was able to lose all his excess weight. And yes, he died—24 years later. And certainly not of starvation!

Myth: Fasting isn't good for women

This myth may stem from a 2012 online article that received 100,000 views and stated that women should not practice fasting for "hormonal reasons," citing "the few studies that exist" pointing to "no." Dr. Fung says nothing could be further from the truth, and in fact, in his practice, he has found that women do much better fasting than do men. Obviously pregnant women and women with eating disorders shouldn't fast. Women (and men) with type 1 diabetes shouldn't fast. Women whose period ceases (usually because they are severely underweight) shouldn't fast. Barring any of these circumstances, fasting is not an issue for women.

Myth: I can't fast because I have non-diabetic hypoglycemia

Non-diabetic hypoglycemia is a very rare condition that occurs if your body can't stabilize your blood levels (this happens if your pancreas produces too much insulin). Non-diabetic hypoglycemia comes in two types:

Reactive hypoglycemia happens a few hours after a heavy meal. Your body produces too much insulin, lowering your blood sugar. With this condition, you're likely at risk of developing diabetes.

Non-reactive hypoglycemia isn't directly related to diet. It may be caused by overconsumption of alcohol, causing your liver to stop producing glucose, side effects of certain medications (often related to kidney failure), severe eating disorders, pregnancy, and disorders of the liver, kidneys, or heart.

If your doctor has said fasting is contraindicated due to non-diabetic reactive hypoglycemia, obviously, follow your doctor's recommendations. However, hypoglycemia is another matter. **Hypoglycemia** is low blood sugar. When you fast, your body has to transition from using glucose for fuel to using ketones. Your cells have to adapt. Sometimes called "keto flu," symptoms may include lightheadedness and headaches. Because our brains rely on glucose almost exclusively, it will experience these symptoms first. Unless you ARE diabetic, this does not pose a health threat. Eating protein will reduce these symptoms, but it's a temporary fix. So, how do you avoid these symptoms?

Instead of heading right into a prolonged fast, gradually transition to ketosis. Start with a 16-hour fast or even 12 hours. Drink water or have bone or vegetable broth if you need to.

Myth: I'll lose muscle

You will not lose muscle. In fact, due to the processes that occur in your body, your fat level will go down, and your lean body muscle will not. Several studies have shown that, compared to calorie-restricted diets, fasting allows you to retain your lean muscle much more effectively. Why would our smart bodies start feasting on our muscle tissue just when we need to go foraging for food? Wouldn't a preferred source of energy be our fat stores?

Myth: Fasting lowers your metabolism

It's true that when we reduce our calories, our bodies adapt, and our metabolism slows to accommodate this new eating plan. We're still getting food on a calorie-restricted diet, so the body doesn't have to run and get food from the deep freezer. It can simply slow down its burn to accommodate the lower levels of glucose it's now receiving. This is the tragedy of calorie-restricted diets, which set us up to fail!

In contrast, as Dr. Fung explains in *The Complete Guide to Fasting*, "… metabolism revs up, not down, during fasting. This makes sense from a survival standpoint. If we do not eat, our bodies use our stored energy as fuel so that we can find more food." This phenomenon is caused by our body's wonderful hormones, which kick in when we fast and make sure we have the energy to go gather and hunt more food; we get that energy from our fat stores.

Myth: Fasting is unhealthy because you'll lose essential nutrients

The sad truth is, we're all likely nutrient-deficient because of the Standard American Diet (SAD diet). Carbohydrates are not essential.[40]

Our bodies need:

---

[40] Dr. Mark Sherwood, "Are Carbohydrates Essential?" Functional Medial Institute (May 25, 2021) https://fmidr.com/carbs-essential/

- Essential fatty acids
- Essential amino acids
- Essential vitamins
- Essential dietary minerals

None of that is provided by carbohydrates.

Some proteins and fats are required for sustaining life because they produce essential amino acids and essential fatty acids. The body does its best to find these for us when we fast. Following a low-carbohydrate diet can help increase our stores of essential amino acids and essential fatty acids, making fasting much, much easier. As mentioned, I also take a food-based multivitamin when I fast—one that isn't going to give me a stomachache! Some of the better ones available are listed here:

- Garden of Life Vitamin Code Women
    - (One goddess I know also swears by their fiber supplement powder)
- MegaFood Women's One Daily (allergen-friendly)
- Nature Made Women's Multivitamin Tablets
- New Chapter Every Woman's One Daily Multivitamin
- New Chapter Multivitamin for Women 50 Plus (contains no iron for those who want to avoid iron)
- Rainbow Lite Women's One Multivitamin

Avoid chewable and gummy-style multivitamins, which often contain sugar.

Fasting Benefits—Beyond Weight Loss

Let's look at a few of the benefits of fasting that go far beyond mere weight loss. Sure, we all want to look good in a bikini, but how about reducing our risk of cancer and Alzheimer's? How about reversing the aging process? Or reducing the risk of stroke and cardiovascular disease?

Let's now look at the bodily processes that occur when we fast for specific periods of time.

Fasting Benefits at Different Durations

Shorter fasts (from 16 hours up to two days)

If you're not used to fasting, for this period of fasting, your energy may feel depleted and you might feel a little "hangry," which is to be expected. In his practice, Dr. Fung says that once a patient is used to intermittent fasting, he rarely suggests a fast for just two days and instead recommends five or more days. Why? Day two is the toughest time, and once you've survived it, you may as well reap the rewards for your perseverance by coasting through another day (or three or five). But know this: Even if you quit at or prior to the two-day mark, you've still reaped many of fasting's benefits.

Mentally, you're exercising your willpower. You're learning to power through those natural urges to eat. Physically, your body is experiencing cleansing and heart health benefits. Fat in your blood starts to disappear as it's metabolized for energy. This promotes a healthy heart and may improve your cholesterol level by boosting HDL levels.

Fasts of 3–7 days

At this stage, ketosis has begun.[41] Ketosis allows your body to burn stored fat (the basement deep freezer) as its primary energy source. Often, you cease feeling hungry or tired. Did you know that when your body receives toxins from external sources or the food you ingest, it shuttles it into fat cells to protect you? Pretty smart, huh? During ketosis, your body can safely expel these toxins from your body as you use up those fat stores. This can have several positive effects, including healing old injuries and clearing up acne and other skin disorders. And here's an incredibly exciting phenomenon, which caused me to do my first five-day fast: Between 72 hours and 120 hours, our bodies begin stem cell regeneration.[42] This has phenomenal health benefits, including antiaging and disease prevention. It has also been suggested as a healing modality to overcome the toxicity of chemotherapy.[43]

---

[41] Ketosis: When your body doesn't have enough carbohydrates to burn for energy, so instead it burns fat, making ketones, which it can use for fuel.

[42] Sarah Knapton, "Fasting for three days can regenerate entire immune system, study finds," Flow In (reprinted Aug 22, 2019) https://www.flowin.com/index.php?page=blog_post&blog_id=79 (reprinted from *The Telegraph*, June 5, 2014)

[43] "Prolonged Fasting reduces IGF-1/PKA to promote hematopoietic stem cell-based regeneration and reverse immunosuppression," National Center for Biotechnology Information (June 5, 2014) https://www.ncbi.nlm.nih.gov/pmc/articles/PMC4102383/

Fasts of 8–15 days

This period begins the "fasting high," similar to the "runner's high" many athletes experience. I felt this myself on my 14-day fast, which I'll cover later. This is also a period of significant healing for the body. Because you're limiting free radicals and oxidative stress, you're encouraging healthy aging and helping to prevent future health problems.

Fasts of 16 days and more

This stage of fasting should be done only under the supervision of a healthcare professional. As we've seen, there isn't much of an upper limit to fasting, with 382 days being the current known record. Don't try to break that record (or even come close to it) without medical supervision! Benefits at this stage are simply more of the same, and you can achieve that with staggered fasting rather than trying to do it all at once.

Nutritional Supplementation During Extended Fasts

If you decide to do a fast of more than 24 hours, it's very important that you ensure your body is getting the nutritional support it needs. Fasting depletes insulin, which is what we want; however, this also causes our bodies to start expelling sodium, potassium, and water. Appropriate supplementation will protect you from some of the more difficult aspects of fasting, such as energy depletion, dehydration, and electrolyte imbalance. It will also help you avoid some of the weight regain that occurs after a fast.

You'll want to ensure you're getting adequate magnesium, potassium, and salt. Some fasting gurus recommend the following amounts:

- **5,000 mg of sodium** – This is about 2 tsp of salt, but take it as Himalayan salt or another marine salt for the extra mineral boost, and take it with water. Table salt won't cut it. I take a pinch at a time then swallow water afterward because I don't mind the taste of salt, and I love my water, but salt water ... yech. If you decide to take bone broth during an extended fast (which I did for several days during my 14-day fast), most will have just under 350 mg of sodium, so you can reduce the amount of other salt you need during the day. Confession: I rarely take as much as 2 tsp of salt during my fasts. That just feels like a lot of salt. You'll find that keto recipes also call for a lot of salt for the same reason. We need that sodium. Of course, if you have reasons to limit your sodium, please discuss options with your doctor.
- **1,000 mg potassium chloride or potassium citrate** – It's important to get the right formulation. When I did my 14-day fast, I didn't know that. I was taking the wrong type, and I was also taking far too little of it.
- **300 mg magnesium malate** – Again, take the right formulation and quantity. I was taking a magnesium potassium blend with only 250 mg of magnesium (the wrong kind) and only 99 mg of potassium (again, the wrong kind). I'm sure some of the issues I

had during my extended fast could have been mitigated or eliminated had I been supplementing appropriately.

You can take these supplements on your eating days as well. Nearly 100% of adults don't get adequate magnesium, and low levels can cause cramping and sleep disorders. As a foot cramp sufferer and occasional insomniac, I'm now a magnesium believer.

Reintroducing Food After an Extended Fast

If you fast for more than 48 hours, it's very important to reintroduce food appropriately and in smaller amounts. Some say that the reintroduction period is as or more important than the fast itself. After one three-day fast, the first thing I put in my mouth was a pumpkin scone and latte. I knew it was wrong, but I did it anyway.

Don't do what I do; do what the experts say. Here's why: Although rare, refeeding syndrome can occur when you immediately introduce some harder-to-digest foods into your body, throwing your electrolytes out of whack. This can cause serious health issues. And you've just cleansed your body and prepared it for great health. Why now throw garbage in?

The reintroduction period should last at least half as long as your fast. So, if you fast for five days, you should be on a careful reintroduction plan for three days. Here's what that looks like for a five-day fast, but if you do an extended fast of say, 10 days, just double up on the day plans (do Day 1 plan for 2 days, Day 2 plan for 2 days, Day 3 plan for 1–2 days).

Day 1

Take in 30-40% of your normal calorie intake. Start with something that will reintroduce good bacteria into your stomach. Examples are sauerkraut juice, pickle juice, kefir, kimchi, apple cider vinegar, or coconut milk yogurt (not commercial yogurt, and only a tablespoon at this point). Coconut water is also great. You can follow that a half hour later with bone broth and later thoroughly steamed veggies (soft enough to mash) or fermented veggies. Be kind to your stomach. You can add ½ tsp of olive oil. Later, you could have a small green salad with some cottage cheese on it (again, only a tablespoon). You can also have green juices containing cucumbers, celery or bok choy, dark leafy greens, herbs (ginger, turmeric, parsley, mint, cilantro), and low glycemic fruits such as lemons and limes.

Day 2

Take in 50% of your normal calorie intake. You can eat raw vegetables and healthy fats (avocado, coconut fats, olives). You can eat healthy (not canned) vegetable soups and stews in bone broth or vegetable broth. If you have steamed veggies, you can add up to 2 tsp of olive oil. On both Days 1 and 2, protein shakes (almond or coconut milk plus bone broth or pea, rice, or hemp protein) are good choices. On Day 2, you can add up to a half-cup of organic berries to your protein shake. You can have a quarter to a half of an avocado. Avocados can help increase the absorption of several antioxidants in salad fixings by a factor of five to 15!

Day 3 and after

You can eat your normal calorie intake if you are still feeling good. Begin to add in some healthy starches and limited quantities of meats and other protein sources, paying attention to your body.

Intermittent fasting is also a great way to come off an extended fast, and, as stated, it can help minimize weight regain.

Autophagy

Autophagy is an outcome of fasting, beginning around 16–24 hours and peaking around 48 hours. Autophagy (it's pronounced like the word esophagus: ah-TOFF-uh-jee) means "self-eating," but don't worry: No cannibals or zombies are involved. Autophagy is the process of cellular cleanup of dangerous and damaged cells—cells that could lead to cancer, inflammation, and other health issues. Think of it as internal exfoliation. Because we've all been conditioned to eat three squares a day (and often several snacks in between), we miss out on this crucial bodily process, and that's a contributing factor to many diseases that are common today but weren't in prior generations.

Another benefit of autophagy is its effect on the skin. It can make it more elastic, allowing it to snap back and adapt to the new weight more quickly. If significant weight loss is required, this is especially helpful in reducing the post-weight loss Shar Pei look.

Knowing how amazing autophagy is for my body, when I'm fasting and start to feel hunger, I tell myself that autophagy is busy doing its job, and so the hunger feeling is a very good sign. My mantra at that time is, "Go, autophagy, go!"

Yes, IF Is for Vegans, Too!

The great thing about intermittent fasting is that you can eat what you want during your feeding time. Choosing mostly healthy food—whether carnivore, omnivore, vegetarian, or full vegan—is all that matters. Supplementing with a full-spectrum food-based multivitamin can help ensure that any essential goodies in your regular diet are accounted for.

CHAPTER 5

Are You Ready? Why Timing Is Crucial to Success

WHEN YOU'RE READY to begin fasting, set yourself up for success. It's crucial that you begin only when you're prepared, because an early failure can leave you thinking "I can't do this." Not true! You're going to struggle. That's part of the process. Push through when it's hard, and the rewards are all there, waiting for you.

Start slowly. Don't start with a full-day or multi-day fast right away, especially if you've never fasted before. And if even 16:8 seems too much for you, try just delaying breakfast by one hour. The next day, try for two. Work up to longer and longer periods between meals.

Time it right. Don't decide to start your fasting program leading up to the holidays, which tend to be full of many food temptations in the high-carb, high-sugar category. After you're used to fasting, you can tackle a big holiday season like a pro, but when you're just starting out, it's best to find a time on the calendar when you'll have the least number of temptations.

Ditch the triggers. Prior to starting your fasting program, get rid of any snacks or foods that you just can't avoid. You're going to need your willpower for other things; be kind to yourself.

> Food is my trigger food.
> ~ Anon

Don't carb load. Just prior to starting your fast, keep carbohydrates to a minimum. This will help your body make and release less insulin, making it easier to tap into fat stores.

Get your sleep. Try to get at least seven hours of sleep each night, and eight is better. Sleep deprivation increases blood sugar levels, which results in more insulin secretion.

Exercise sensibly. If you regularly get some form of exercise, you can choose to continue this while you fast, but maybe take it back a notch. Some athletes find that fasting gives them such great energy they're able to exercise at a higher level of exertion, and they recover much more quickly. But don't test this, especially when you're first starting out. That said, overall, getting some form of regular cardiovascular exercise is good for you and can increase the benefits you gain from fasting because it causes your body to use sugars immediately. This reduces the need for insulin and reduces fat storage. Lack of activity does just the opposite. Weight training can increase lean muscle, which increases metabolism and strengthens muscles, ligaments, and even our bones, which can help prevent injury.

If you regularly prepare food for others, cook twice as much, half as often. Prepare twice as much food as you need when cooking so you can freeze half. Then, on days you don't intend to eat, you'll have an easy meal that won't require preparation. There's a great book called *Frozen Assets: How to Cook for a Day and Eat for a Month* that you may want to check out.

Avoid creamers and sweeteners in your coffee. While it's fine to drink black coffee or tea when fasting, don't add sweeteners (even artificial sweeteners) to your beverages. Avoid soda, even diet soda. If you must have cream in your coffee, you can add full-fat cream (it has the fat without the carbs) but not half and half, and try to limit it to 1–2 tsp a day. (That's not much; I've measured it out, and it doesn't change the color much, so it's probably easiest to avoid it entirely.) For a treat, try sprinkling some Ceylon cinnamon into your coffee.

Take a pinch of salt if you need it. If you feel like you're getting weak, add a pinch of pink Himalayan salt to your water or just take a pinch on your tongue. It will give you a slight boost of energy.

Stay well hydrated. Keep a glass of water at your side and sip on it throughout the day, refilling as needed.

Plan your "break-the-fast" meal in advance. Know what you're going to eat when you break your fast, and if needed, prepare it ahead of time so you can just eat without being in the kitchen around all those other temptations. How many times do we eat when preparing food?!

How to Eat When You Do Eat

During your eating time, try to eat low carb and high fat as much as possible. This may feel foreign to you, but it can really help your body fat adapt, which will make fasting so much easier. I've provided some of my favorite low-carb, high-fat recipes in the back of this book, but once you get used to eating this way, you'll find you can easily modify any meal to accommodate a lower-carb eating plan.

For instance, when I make my son spaghetti, I use marinara sauce without sugar, add grass-fed ground beef with herbs and spices, and serve his over pasta, while I eat mine over zoodles (spiralized zucchini noodles) or salad greens. It's just as delicious, even more so, because I can add a glass of wine and still be in good carb territory. When I make "High Nachos," a favorite in our household, I skip the refried beans for me and put the seasoned beef over a bed of greens with just a few crumbled tortilla chips. I use salsa for dressing and add a sprinkle of shredded cheese and cilantro. It's like a delicious and healthy taco salad!

And speaking of vegetables, I learned this trick online: Make sure that vegetables are half of your meal (meaning greens, green beans, broccoli, cauliflower, Brussels sprouts, not corn or potatoes). If everyone did this one thing, we'd all be much healthier. On days I eat breakfast, I'll often make myself a veggie frittata or a quiche muffin loaded with shredded veggies (I've shared these recipes in the back). I delay breakfast until 10:30 or 11 a.m., and I skip lunch, but we eat dinner quite early in my house (due to my son, who gets ravenous if food isn't on the table by 4 p.m.). So, I've finished eating by 5 p.m. most days, and I rarely snack afterward unless I'm feeling particularly indulgent, in which case I may have some popcorn with plenty of butter! I make it the old-fashioned way—in a pan, on top of the stove. Although the cancer risks once attributed to microwave popcorn have apparently been eliminated, I try to ensure everything we eat is as natural as possible. (And we don't have a microwave, so that's not an option.)

> Avocado oil is a heart-healthy oil high in oleic acid, which is an unsaturated fat. It contains vitamin E and also helps the body absorb other fat-soluble vitamins. Avocado oil is a good source of monounsaturated fat, which has been linked to reducing LDL cholesterol and increasing HDL cholesterol.
>
> **WebMD**

Substitute cauliflower rice in your rice dishes. If you've never tried it, trust me: It's quite good. I've tried making my own (by ricing, dicing, or carefully shredding cauliflower), but it's available in bags in the frozen food aisle, and that's usually what I use.

Add 2–3 tablespoons of healthy fat to your evening meal. This can be olive oil drizzled over your salad, for instance, or half an avocado. This will help keep your blood sugar level steady overnight. **Note:** Healthy fats are avocado, nuts, olive oil, avocado oil, ghee, butter, and natural nut butter. They are not canola oil, "vegetable oil," margarine, or shortening. Also, olive oil is great for salads, not so great for cooking. For cooking, use avocado oil, coconut oil, or MCT oil. Olive oil gives off toxic smoke when heated, and heating it destroys many of its health benefits.

Try to eat your last food well before bedtime. Eating just prior to bedtime, especially carbs, causes you to store fat while sleeping. **Fact:** We burn most of our fat while sleeping unless we overwhelm our body with sugars. You'll lose an important opportunity to burn fat if you eat too close to bedtime. Some fasting experts say the best eating window for weight loss is between 8 a.m. and 3 p.m., or even 8 a.m. to 2 p.m. That's not feasible for most of us. Do what fits into your lifestyle.

Don't beat yourself up if you decide to eat on a day or time when you planned to fast. Beating yourself up is the very definition of self-defeating behavior. No matter what Yoda said, trying *is* doing. (Yoda is an unattractive, short, fictional alien, and you don't have to listen to him.) Love yourself for trying. Trying is a win—congratulate yourself for winning! Then decide how you can set yourself up for an even bigger win next time.

CHAPTER 6

The Keto Connection

WANT TO FAST WHILE YOU'RE EATING? Eat keto. Many of the same results that can be had from fasting (fat loss, weight loss, health benefits) are also realized with the high-fat, low-carb ketogenic diet. In fact, many people combine these two approaches for a sustainable healthy lifestyle.

How Keto Works

Ketosis is a metabolic state in which your body uses fat for fuel instead of glucose. Sound familiar? It should. Other than fasting, one way to get into a ketogenic state is by significantly reducing your carb intake, such as with a ketogenic diet. For most women, that means no more than 20 grams of carbs per day, and for reference, a medium apple has 25 grams of carbohydrates.

On keto, you also limit your protein, fueling your body with predominantly healthy fats. With a keto diet, the breakdown is around 75% fat, 20% protein, and 5% carbohydrates. Why limit protein? Protein can be converted into glucose when you take in more than moderate amounts.

Ketosis allows you to eat and lose weight without counting calories. In 2020, my cousin lost 100 pounds on keto, and he's kept it off. He also incorporated some intermittent fasting.

My Own Keto Experiment

At one point, I went strictly keto for two months. I also had my 19-year-old son on keto, and although he's a particular eater, he loved the foods: meats, fats, some nice vegetables. Very little fruit or sweets, however, so I had to go to great lengths to find ways to keep his sweet tooth satisfied without sugar. I bought several keto cookbooks and cleaned out my pantry of carbs. I bought ingredients that had never been past my kitchen door before: MCT oil, monk fruit sweetener, xylitol, coconut flour, Swerve sweetener, stevia-sweetened chocolate chips, nutritional yeast, cans of coconut milk (for keto milkshakes), paleo turkey bacon, and sugar-free ham purchased online (most ham has some sugar added during its processing).

Our results were that I lost about 12 pounds over two months, and my son lost 36! For the record, although my son and I both had some weight to lose, I put us on keto for another health reason relating to my son. It was an experiment, and, on that level, it failed, but we both lost significant weight and had no health issues. In fact, I tend to suffer from digestion issues, and I had none while I was on keto, so I still do mostly keto, but I can't be that strict. I love food freedom too much.

We did have two incidents on keto. Potassium levels can get dangerously low—something I didn't know when we started. One day, while shopping at Whole Foods, I felt as though I needed to slide to the floor. I felt totally fine, great even—I just needed to lie down suddenly. It happened in an aisle, and again as I was checking out. I learned then about the need to supplement with potassium, and we began taking it and had no further incidents-- except one.

> Both total fasting and a ketogenic diet lead to an accelerated sodium excretion that increases water and salt loss through the urine. If this lost sodium is not replaced, the resulting deficit [tells] the body to conserve this vital element. The kidneys will reabsorb sodium to reduce its excretion ... this process comes at the price of increased potassium excretion.
>
> **VirtaHealth.com**

My son stayed with his dad one weekend, and I prepared and sent all his keto meals with him, but I neglected to pack the potassium. Not realizing that, I picked him up from his dad's that Sunday, and we went directly to an outdoor event—a Hawaiian festival in a nearby town. We parked a couple of blocks away and walked to the fair. I'd brought my son's water bottle for him, and he was sipping on it as we walked. At one point, he was drinking out of the bottle and walking at the same time, and he started to stumble. I caught his arm, righted him, and teased him about being clumsy, and we kept walking. A few steps later, though, not drinking from the bottle, he stumbled again. "Are you okay?" I asked. "I'm fine," he insisted. "I'm just really tired." I knew then what was happening, and I tried to get him to a gazebo where I hoped there was a bench, but as we approached it, he went down. I called for a medic, asked for electrolytes, and then ran for the car. By the time I returned with the car, he was already feeling better, and as we drove away, he said he wanted to stop by the library to pick up a book he had on hold. So, we went to the library. I kept a good eye on him, but he was fine.

Like I said, I still do modified keto, and I take my potassium. My son, however, eats whatever the heck he wants (luckily, he makes mostly healthy choices), but we're talking *quantity*, girlfriend. He's also managed to keep off most of the weight he lost during our keto experiment. Lucky devil.

Keto Shade

There have been some reports that keto is an unhealthy way to lose weight and carries risk. The *U.S. News & World Report*, for instance, called it one of the top unhealthy diet trends.

Do your own research, but I'm a keto believer. I'm just not a keto poster child because I prefer to have more flexibility in the food I eat. I'd rather choose *when* I eat than be limited in *what* I eat, within reason.

CHAPTER 7

Help for Carb and Sugar Addicts

AS ANY GRADUATE OF A 12-STEP PROGRAM will tell you, half the battle of conquering an addiction is admitting you have one. I could write an entire book on carb and sugar addiction, and how dangerous they are, but those have already been written. Two books I highly recommend are *The Case Against Sugar,* by Gary Taubes, and *Wheat Belly*, by William Davis. The first will help you understand that sugar is a poison—one we gladly ingest and feed to our children. The second will help you understand that just because something is whole grain doesn't make it healthy or good for us.

Please keep in mind that the type of addiction I'm discussing here does not compare with heroin or cocaine addiction, though there are some similarities and some people will swear it does. Only you can know how big of a hold these "substances" have on you. But be cautious about programs that are restrictive in the extreme. I looked into Bright Line because a goddess told me it was her solution. She felt intermittent fasting didn't meet her needs because during her feeding window her food addictions were too hard to control.

I'm not discounting anyone's personal experience with food. You know you best. I distinctly remember a time when my youngest son, as a toddler, was exposed to Goldfish crackers for the first time. We'd just stopped by to drop off something at the house of an acquaintance, and he saw the crackers and ate several. Then several more in rapid succession. He was in what I can only describe as a trance—completely unaware of his surroundings and frenzied. It was embarrassing, but mostly it frightened me. I later discovered that he had a gluten intolerance, and we often crave what we shouldn't have. (My son is mostly gluten-free now, as am I, and when he does have gluten on occasion, it's not an issue.)

So specific foods can be a problem for some of us, and I hope I've made it clear that, although we really *can* have whatever we want during our feeding window, for the best results and our overall health, we should eat healthy most of the time. However, the title of this book is *Goddesses Don't Diet* for a reason. Haven't we been held prisoner long enough by food-diet-weight-loss-fitness tyrants? I don't think we should let anyone dictate what we do with our own bodies. If you have a severe addiction to any type of food, that's something to take up with your medical professional. Absent that, listen to your body, and do what's right for you.

If you're intrigued, research Bright Line for yourself, but be sure to check out an article on abbylangernutrition.com titled "Bright Line Eating Review: A Shame-Filled Marketing Monster." And be leery of any program that's too restrictive. I've mentioned keto, which for most of us is too restrictive as a lifestyle. I use keto principles (low carb, healthy fats) but I don't even follow that all the time and I don't box myself into a corner. That's not sustainable. Fasting *is* because the flexibility and freedom is built into it. You can use it when you want as you want.

Now, let's look at sugar and carb addiction. Notice that you never hear anyone complaining about fat or protein addiction. There's a very good reason for that. Fats and proteins don't have the same effect on our bodies or our brains.

If, like me, you'd rather have a bag of tortilla chips than a brownie, you're probably a carb addict. If you'd rather have the brownie, sugar may be your drug of choice. The two are closely related, however, and as we've learned, carbs turn into glucose in our bodies, so we carbaholics may as well have eaten sugar to begin with.

The relationship between carb and sugar addiction is obvious when you think about it: When sugar addicts eliminate sugar, they often have intense cravings for carbohydrates. And we carb lovers will rarely turn down that brownie once the chips are gone. Usually, both addictions happily (if unhealthily) cohabitate. My sweet tooth may play second fiddle to my carb monster, but it's there.

Our bodies were designed to seek out carbs and sugar; these provide a quick burst of energy and helped our ancestors store body fat for the times when food wasn't always available. But we no longer need that source of quick fuel, and it's killing us—shortening our lifespan, adding excess weight, and increasing our risk for disease.

> Sugar does induce the same responses in the region of the brain known as the "reward center"... as do nicotine, cocaine, heroin, and alcohol.
>
> **Gary Taube, *The Case Against Sugar***

Eliminating table sugar, high-fructose corn syrup, and white flour can cause withdrawal symptoms, and it may be responsible for what's been termed as "keto flu." Those on a ketogenic diet eliminate sugar and most carbs. The withdrawal period may last only a day or two, but it's significant. Sugar causes an opioid reaction in our brain, impacting our pleasure center. The cravings we get when we withdraw from sugar may be attributed to that.

If we don't make it past the withdrawal period, it can lead to binge eating on sugar and carbs, after which we feel remorse and guilt. How do we feel "good" again? We feed those opioids more carbs and sugar. And the cycle continues.

Breaking the cycle requires discipline and time. And it also requires reading labels. Some of the most innocuous seeming products contain added sugar: ketchup, salad dressings, lightly processed ham, bacon, sausage, and most processed foods.

When my son had the "I'm fine; I'm just really tired" crash at the park and I called a medic over, I knew he needed electrolytes. I asked the medic for some Gatorade or other electrolyte drink. He brought over electrolyte powder, mixed it with some bottled water, and tipped the cup back for my son. "Not too much," I warned. "He's been off sugar, and I don't want him to get sick."

"Off sugar?! Why? He *needs* sugar!" the medic said, alarmed. Our bodies do not need sugar. They think they do, however.

In *The Case Against Sugar*, Taubes writes that the more we use sugar, the less dopamine is produced naturally in our brain, and the more habituated our brain cells become to the dopamine it does produce, resulting in a decrease in the number of dopamine receptors. I don't know about you, but I'd like to keep as many dopamine receptors as I can.

Overconsumption of sugar is literally killing us. A study by the American Heart Association (AHA) in March 2013 attributed 180,000 deaths worldwide to the consumption of sugary beverages. And a study by the American Medical Association in January of that same year found that fructose (e.g., table sugar, high fructose corn syrup) stimulates our appetite and causes us to eat more. Ditto with artificial sweeteners.[44]

---

[44] How to Break the Sugar Habit – and Help Your Health in the Process, July 1,

To kick the sugar and carb addiction, don't have too many temptations in your house, particularly not sweet treats or other nonhealthy carbs. Indulge in those on special occasions only. At Halloween, I usually give out Butterfingers and candy corn because I dislike them intensely. If I were to buy Reese's or Hershey's with almonds or Almond Joys and had any leftovers, they might not see November 1.

Buy unsweetened versions of yogurt, oatmeal, and iced tea and only add a small amount of sugar, weaning yourself off it over time. I usually take my coffee black, but when I visited a friend recently, her daughter kept a mocha flavored Coffee Mate creamer in the refrigerator for coffee. I found myself adding that to my first cup in the morning. Then I came to rely on it for my second cup as well. As soon as I got home, I was able to kick that habit because it wasn't right there in the fridge for me to use.

Avoid soda. I stopped drinking soda (even diet soda) more than a decade ago. However, I recently discovered Zevia, which is a 0-calorie soda sweetened with stevia. I usually find stevia bitter, but I don't taste it in this soda. If you're a soda fan, you might want to switch to this brand. My son likes the root beer flavor, and I prefer the grapefruit flavor. It's believed that stevia doesn't increase blood sugar, and I've not found that it leads to cravings of sugary snacks. And stevia won't break a fast, at least according to some nutritionists. If I need a treat when doing an extended fast, or even an alternate day fast, I'll sometimes have a Zevia. It's a nice treat

---

2013, Harvard Health Publishing, https://www.health.harvard.edu/staying-healthy/how-to-break-the-sugar-habit-and-help-your-health-in-the-process

instead a glass of wine when I'm reading in bed at the end of the day.

If it's carbs, not sugar, that's the issue, or if you're a dual addict like me, the best way to kick a carb addiction to the curb (*kerb*, if you're a British goddess) is to start with keto. You'll find that the high fat content is very satisfying, and once you're "fat adapted," you mostly lose your craving for carbs. Even if, like me, you decide keto is too restrictive to do long-term, if you stay on it for even a few weeks, you'll develop the practice of not centering meals around carbs.

What Is Fat Adaptation?

As we've covered, carbs aren't the only fuel our bodies can run on; they can also run on fat. But we have to train our bodies to use fat for fuel by doing some work on our metabolic engine. When our body becomes a fat burner, this is called being fat adapted. Conversion from running on carbs to running on fat requires time. Our body has to create new fat burning pathways and enzymes.

Until you're fat adapted, your body is going to tell you to eat sugar and carbs, because it doesn't yet know there's another perfectly good fuel available. It will tell you to feed it sugar and carbs by making you think you're sick. This can manifest as tiredness, shakiness, and cloudy thinking. Consider this a good sign! You're in transition, and you may need a few days, even a week or two, for your body to adjust, but it will adjust because it must adjust. Be patient; it's learning a new trick, and once it's learned, it's going to be a new fat burning machine. For more on this, see the YouTube video "Common Traps for New Low Carb Dieters," by Dr. Becky Gillaspy (her website is drbeckyfitness.com). In the video, she also discusses the mental transition that must take place. Well worth a watch, and she has a lovely, calm demeanor I think you'll appreciate.

To ease the shift from high carb to low carb, there are some wonderful alternatives to refined carbs now—riced cauliflower for rice, zoodles for pasta, cauliflower crust for pizza. Many restaurants offer lettuce wraps in lieu of the bun or bread for your sandwich. I've been low carb for so long now that the idea of eating an entire bagel seems outrageous to me. And I used to think they were healthy! I still have my carb triggers though—tortilla chips are my weakness. It's the salty crunch more than the carbs, though, that gets me.

> Sugar is the most inflammatory food there is. Because inflammation is so destructive, your body must direct resources to deal with it. Resources that it would otherwise use to run your immune system.
>
> **Dr. Becky Gillaspy**

Look for foods low on the glycemic index. The glycemic index is a way to measure how much a specific food can increase your blood sugar levels. Remember that carbs may go in as carbs, but our body treats them like glucose. And not all carbs are created equal. Sweet potatoes are a better alternative than white potatoes, but they still have plenty of carbs (16.8 g vs 20.4 g in their 3.5 oz. white cousin).

Sweet potatoes, however, have more fiber and are lower on the glycemic index, despite containing more sugar.

Why do our bodies crave sugar and carbs when they're not good for us? Shouldn't we have evolved to only crave what our bodies need? The answer lies in our brain's dopamine response. When we eat sugar (or carbs that turn into glucose), our brain produces huge surges of dopamine. This dopamine flooding is similar to how our brain reacts when we ingest heroin and cocaine. Scientists believe that, due to food scarcity, our bodies adapted over time to seek foods high in calories that are quickly converted to energy in order to survive. But now can get a Frappuccino on every corner, and our bodies haven't caught up yet with this change. Our brains still perceive sugar as beneficial and produce gobs of dopamine when we eat sugary, high-calorie foods. Constantly feeding this need feeds cravings and even withdrawal when we cut it out of our diets. Other laboratory studies have shown that a daily dose of sugar keeps us hooked. The more we have, the more we want. So, keeping sugar at bay, minimizing its intake, helps us maintain control. An occasional treat? Sure! A regular "fix"? Not so much.

Dr. Gillaspy recommends having a high fat salad each day as you wean yourself from sugar. The greens provide volume and the fat (sliced boiled eggs, avocado, olive oil, nuts, and cheese) can help keep hunger at bay. She also says for any eating plan to be sustainable for life it must be the three Es: It must be *enjoyable* (allowing freedom). It must be *effective* (this means you must have continual evidence that it's working) and it must be *easy* to follow. If you find that cutting out sugar and refined carbs is too hard for you, take it in stages. Try cutting back before cutting out.

CHAPTER 8

Sleep, Water, and Exercise

NO, FASTING IS NOT EASY, but it does get easier, and it's one of the best things you can do for your health, weight, and overall wellbeing.

Three other healthy choices you can make that can also increase your fasting success are getting adequate sleep, drinking plenty of water, and getting appropriate exercise.

Sleep Like a Baby

Getting regular adequate sleep is something too few of us do. According to the American Sleep Apnea Association (ASAA), 70% of Americans report that they get inadequate sleep at least one night per month; 11% of Americans report that they regularly get inadequate sleep. Per the ASAA, sleep is "as vital as the air we breathe and the food we eat."[45]

Matthew Walker, PhD, is a professor of neuroscience and psychology at UC Berkley, the director of its Sleep and Neuroimaging Lab, and a former professor of psychiatry at Harvard University. In his book, *Why We Sleep*, he writes, "Sleeping less than six or seven hours a night demolishes your immune system, more than doubling your risk of cancer. It also disrupts blood sugar levels so profoundly that you would be classified as pre-diabetic." In addition, he writes that *short sleeping* increases risk for coronary artery blockage and hardening, which can lead to cardiovascular disease, stroke, and congestive heart failure.[46]

> I love to sleep. Do you? Isn't it great? It really is the best of both worlds. You get to be alive and unconscious.
>
> **Rita Rudner,
> American Comedian**

Remember ghrelin, the hormone that puts the grr in hunger, and leptin, the hormone that signals the "I'm full" feeling? Short sleep reduces leptin and increases ghrelin. As Dr. Walker writes in his book, this is like "being punished twice for the same offense."[47] And importantly, Dr. Walker reports that when we don't get adequate

---

[45] SleepHealth.org (May 25, 2021) https://www.sleephealth.org/sleep-health/the-state-of-sleephealth-in-america/

[46] Walker, Matthew, PhD, *Why We Sleep: Unlocking the Power of Sleep and Dreams*

[47] Ibid

sleep, the extra calories we eat while we're awake longer far outweigh the few extra calories we burn by being up and at 'em a little longer.

Three decades of research have shown that the same people who sleep less are the same individuals who are more likely to be overweight or obese. When we're not getting enough sleep, our bodies become "especially stingy," says Dr. Walker, "about giving up fat." Instead, muscle mass is depleted, and fat is maintained. To sum up his work on sleep deprivation as it relates to weight loss, short sleep as is commonly seen in first-world countries, and does the following:

- Increases hunger and appetite
- Compromises impulse control within the brain
- Increases food consumption, especially high calorie foods
- Decreases feelings of food satisfaction after eating
- Prevents effective weight loss when dieting

On the flip side, studies have shown that adequate sleep repairs the communication pathway between deep brain areas that lead to overindulgence and restores our system of impulse control.[48]

Caffeine can disrupt our sleep, reports Dr. Walker, particularly as we age, because the older we are, the longer it takes our brain and body to remove caffeine from our system.

---

[48]ibid

Alcohol may sedate us out of wakefulness, but it does not induce natural sleep. It fragments sleep and suppresses REM sleep (Walker). Poor sleep and medicated sleep do not promote the immune repair that takes place during in natural sleep.

High carb diets can decrease the amount of deep sleep we get.

Exercise during the day can help you sleep, but try to fit it in at least two to three hours before bed because it revs up your metabolism, and you don't need that when you're trying to get to sleep.

You should also **avoid electronics** at least an hour before sleep, more if possible. Reading is fine, but not on your electronic devices. Blue light decreases the body's natural melatonin production by 25–50%, and those effects can linger for days after ceasing! This is bad news for us who do a lot of work online, so consider using eyeglasses that block blue light. The verdict is still out on their effectiveness, so try it for yourself and see if it works for you. Software is also available to desaturate blue LED light from computers, smartphones, and tablets as the evening progresses.

Use **blackout curtains** (or an eye mask) to ensure your bedroom is as dark as possible. If insomnia is a significant issue for you, the National Sleep Foundation (at thensf.org) has a list of qualified therapists.

The National Institute on Aging offers the following 12 tips for healthy sleep:

1. Stick to a sleep schedule. Go to bed and wake up at the same time.
2. Exercise for 30 minutes most days, but not later than 2–3 hours before bedtime.
3. Avoid caffeine and nicotine at least 8 hours before bed.
4. Avoid alcohol before bed. It harms REM sleep and causes wakefulness.
5. Avoid large meals at night and too many fluids.
6. Avoid medications that may impact sleep.
7. Don't take naps after 3 p.m.
8. Relax before bed. Read, listen to music.
9. Take a hot bath before bed. It relaxes you, and the drop in body temperature after getting out can help you relax and slow down so you're more ready for sleep.
10. Have a dark, cool, gadget-free bedroom.
11. During the day, get outside for 30–60 minutes in the sun first thing in the morning. This helps set your circadian rhythm.
12. Don't lie in bed awake. If you've been trying to sleep for more than 20 minutes, get up and do something relaxing so you're not anxious about not sleeping.[49]

Water: Tonic for the Goddess

Water helps flush out fat and toxins, transports nutrients throughout our body, clears our skin, and flushes bacteria from our

---

[49] "A Good Night's Sleep" National Institute on Aging (May 25, 2021) https://www.nia.nih.gov/health/good-nights-sleep

bladders. It also aids digestion, prevents constipation, normalizes blood pressure, stabilizes our heartbeat, cushions our joints, protects our organs and tissues, regulates our body temperature, and helps maintain our electrolyte balance.

But who needs it?

Common laments in the weight loss community are: "I have to get my water in," or "I hate drinking all that water," or "I'm not really a water drinker." We usually hear that we should drink eight eight-ounce glasses of water a day, but that may not be true for all of us. In fact, Harvard Health suggests that four to six glasses a day is fine.[50] Still other studies say you should aim for between half an ounce of water to an ounce of water for every pound you weigh. For instance, a 120-pound person should drink between 60 and 120 ounces.

> Drinking water is like washing out your insides. The water will cleanse the system, fill you up, decrease your caloric load, and improve the function of all your tissues.
>
> **Kevin R. Stone, MD**

Some people must limit their water intake for medical reasons. If you're not one of those people, aim for eight glasses of water a day. If your pee turns clear, you've had enough. It should be a lemony yellow, not dark yellow or orange.

---

[50] "How Much Water Should You Drink?" Harvard Health Publishing (March 25, 2020) https://www.health.harvard.edu/staying-healthy/how-much-water-should-you-drink

Because we normally get some of our water from food, when you fast, you'll need to replace what you're missing with another glass or two.

If you exercise and sweat water off, you'll need to drink more water. (Usually, you'll want to drink more water because exercise makes you thirsty.)

Ways to enjoy water more

You can drink water cold or at room temperature. I prefer room temperature unless it's hot out. You can also drink hot water or substitute herbal tea for a glass of water. You can infuse your water with slices or sprigs of the following fruits, vegetables, and herbs:

- Lime
- Lemon
- Orange
- Cucumber
- Mint leaves, basil, ginger, rosemary, cilantro
- Frozen berries, used in lieu of ice cubes
- Pineapple
- Melon

You can also drink sparkling water or seltzer for a pop of fizz. You can freeze slices of mandarin oranges and use them as ice cubes. Just don't eat those ice cubes on fasting days.

Exercise: The 5% Solution

We all know exercise is important, and yet very few of us get enough of it or the right type of it consistently, this author included. When it comes to weight loss, what we put in our mouths (or don't) is 95% of the equation; exercise is the other 5%. But far beyond weight loss, there are many health reasons to exercise.

In addition to regular cardiovascular exercise, such as walking, jogging, or running, weight-bearing exercise is crucial. Every pound of muscle you carry equals 50 calories burned, so weight resistance should be part of your exercise plan. Aim for 150 minutes of exercise each week, and make sure that you do weight-bearing exercise twice per week.

Harvard Medical School lists the following exercises as best for overall health.[51]

Strength Training

As mentioned, toned muscles burn calories. Strength training can also protect our bones and prevent injury. Simple strength training exercises that require no equipment include pushups, sit-ups, yoga, squats, planks, burpees, pull-ups, and Pilates. If you'd like to try arm weights, there is a great YouTube video called "Get Madonna's Arms with This 10-Minute Workout" by Pop Sugar, which I love. You use three and five-pound dumbbells, alternating between these for each type of exercise. You'll be sore at first (pace yourself), but after a

---

[51] "5 of the best exercises you can ever do," Harvard Health Publishing (July 7, 2020) https://www.health.harvard.edu/staying-healthy/5-of-the-best-exercises-you-can-ever-do

couple of weeks of twice-weekly workouts, seeing the immediate improvement in arm tone will help you, like Madonna, get Into the Groove.

Swimming

Swimming is easy on your joints, which is great for those with arthritis and joint pain, and it can be a mood lifter. Water aerobics is an option as well, which can help you both burn calories and get toned.

Tai Chi

You may have seen practitioners of this Chinese martial art in a nearby park. Tai chi has been called "meditation in motion" and is basically a series of graceful movements, each transitioning smoothly into the next. Tai chi can improve both fitness level and balance, which is important as we age. Its meditative aspects can also improve mental state and brain health.

Walking

Walking can help you lose weight, improve cholesterol levels, strengthen bones, keep blood pressure in check, lift your mood, and lower your risk for diabetes and heart disease. When the weather is bad, I'll often pop in one of Leslie Sansone's walking videos. They're great exercise and help tone many muscles you don't usually use when walking.

Kegels

Surprised to see this on Harvard's list? Apparently, Kegel exercises can help us strengthen pelvic floor muscles, which support the bladder, helping to prevent incontinence. Kegels aren't just for women, either; men can benefit as well. To do a Kegel, squeeze the muscles you would use to prevent yourself from passing urine or gas. Hold for two to three seconds, then release. Repeat 10 times and do a set four to five times a day.

Frankly, I'm surprised Harvard didn't include a few other forms of exercise on its list. I'll remedy that now.

HIIT

High-intensity interval training involves repeated, short intervals of full-out exercise followed by periods of recovery at a moderate pace. This can be sprinting when you're out for a jog or increasing your pace on the treadmill or stationary bike to maximum capability for a period of time, then leveling off, then repeating. By forcing your body to switch between two very different states, you improve its cardio conditioning. And bonus: It improves insulin sensitivity and blood pressure. It can also burn more calories than a lower-intensity workout and is a great form of exercise when you're short on time.

Rebounding

Rebounding is my go-to exercise, and I absolutely love it. Rebounding is working out on a mini trampoline, or rebounder. NASA didn't invent rebounding, but it did find that it was the "most efficient, effective exercise yet devised."[52] NASA used it to get its astronauts back in shape after "deconditioning" due to the weightlessness of space. In fact, it was found to be better for that purpose than was running. Rebounding is gentle on the joints, yet it helps work muscles in the legs, increases endurance, and strengthens bones. It has also been shown to positively impact blood sugar markers.

In addition, it boosts balance and coordination and supports pelvic floor health. Each time you bounce, your entire body pulls up, which can strengthen pelvic floor muscles. And it's the only exercise I know of that's both easy on the joints and helps improve the lymphatic and immune systems. The vertical bouncing, as opposed to horizontal movements while running, promotes drainage and circulation of lymphatic fluids, draining toxins and other buildup, which allows our immune system to function optimally.

> Without adequate movement, the cells are left stewing in their own waste products and starving for nutrients, a situation that contributes to arthritis, cancer and other degenerative diseases. ... [R]ebounding is reported to increase lymph flow by 15 to 30 times. Also, bones become stronger with exercise.
>
> **Wellbeing Journal**

---

[52] "NASA Studies Rebounding," Rebound Therapy (May 25, 2021) https://www.reboundtherapy.org/edu/root/rebound%20therapy%20study%20and%20research/NASA_Studies_Rebounding.pdf

When I rebound, I put on my iPod, tucking it into a pocket or otherwise attaching it to my clothing, put in my earbuds, and play some great music. I aim to work out for 6–8 songs, which is usually 22–30 minutes. But I don't just stand there and bounce. I jog for one song, and for the next song, I do high knees. Then I repeat. I believe this is a better workout than simply bouncing, which I would find boring for that length of time.

You can spend nearly $400 on a mini trampoline or around $40. I've had both, and they both do the trick.

Yoga

There's just something about yoga. It helps us create a closer relationship with our bodies. It's self-care and self-love in one non-judgmental package. It's great for conditioning our core, improving our balance, and strengthening our muscles. It's also good for you mentally and spiritually. I did prenatal yoga when I was pregnant with my first child. It was very relaxing and gave me the inner peace to prepare for what would be the first of two natural childbirths.

One of my favorite yoga DVDs is Mandy Ingber's *Yogalosophy*, which combines yoga with toning exercises. And I don't do it nearly enough.

Frequent and Small

If you're like me and have a sedentary job and find yourself working late into the night on projects sitting in front of a computer, getting adequate exercise can be a challenge. But you don't have to do it all at once. Taking frequent breaks to stretch, walk, or do some form of exercise is just as beneficial—perhaps more so—than a longer session. Why? Sitting too long is very bad for our health. It can cause many issues, including muscle atrophy, weight gain, hip and back problems, anxiety, and depression. It can also increase our risk for cancer, diabetes, and heart disease, not to mention varicose veins, deep vein thrombosis, and stiff shoulders and neck. And besides all those health issues, it can also cause you to have a flat butt (the worst!).

Although I purchased a standup desk, I find I get busy and focused and don't use it as much as I should. One thing that has worked is building in an exercise break every hour. I created an exercise checklist and have it on the bulletin board by my work desk. I check off exercises each hour, which gets me up and off my flattening butt.

Here's my list:

- 8 a.m.: 25 squats
- 9 a.m.: 2 songs (I walk for the length of two songs, which I play on my iPod)
- 10 a.m.: pushups
- 11 a.m.: 2 songs
- 12 p.m.: HIIT (my 10-minute rebounding session)
- 1 p.m.: 2 songs
- 2 p.m.: 10 lunges (each leg)
- 3 p.m.: 2 songs
- 4 p.m.: grab bag

When I lived on Maui, the grab bag was a walk to the beach (don't hate me; I no longer live there). Now it might be a treadmill session, another set of squats, or whatever I feel like doing (and often, it's putting dinner on the table).

Meditation: Train Your Brain, Train Your Bod

While not physical exercise, meditation does provide brain exercise, which can stimulate physical changes to neural fibers. This can have benefits for the body as well. Scans have shown that meditation can rewire the brain, and it has been used effectively to treat depression and anxiety.[53] A study at UCLA found that long-term meditators had better-preserved brains than non-meditators as they aged, so it also has antiaging benefits.[54] There are many ways—and no wrong ways—to meditate, so select the method that's best for you. Some combine more than one type of meditation, and each generally starts with one or three cleansing breaths to prepare for the meditation.

---

[53] "Mindfulness meditation: A mental workout to benefit the brain," Harvard University Science in the News blog article (April 15, 2013) https://sitn.hms.harvard.edu/flash/2013/mindfulness-meditation-a-mental-workout-to-benefit-the-brain/#:~:text=Such%20benefits%20may%20seem%20far,widespread%20ramifications%20for%20the%20body

[54] Alice G. Walton, "7 Ways Meditation Can Actually Change the Brain," *Forbes* (Feb 9, 2015) https://www.forbes.com/sites/alicegwalton/2015/02/09/7-ways-meditation-can-actually-change-the-brain/?sh=5459228d1465

Mindfulness

Mindfulness is simply paying attention to your thoughts as they pass, merely as observation and without judgment. You can focus on your breath if that's helpful.

Spiritual

Spiritual meditation is often done as a religious practice, either at home or in a place of worship, and may incorporate essential oils to heighten the experience. Prayer is a form of meditation for many.

Focused

With focused meditation, you concentrate using one of the five senses. You might count mala or rosary beads, listen to a gong, stare at a candle flame, or focus on your breath. As your mind begins to wander, bring it back to the object of focus.

Movement

Tai chi, qigong, and nature walks are all forms of movement meditation.

Mantra

With this type of meditation, you select a mantra and say it softly or at full volume. A familiar example is "Ohm." The mantra can be used with many of these meditation types.

Transcendental meditation

This type of more structured meditation uses a mantra or series of words specific to the practitioner.

Progressive relaxation

With progressive relaxation meditation, you tense, then relax one muscle group at a time, often starting with the feet and moving up the body. This can be effective in helping to unwind before bed.

Loving-kindness

Loving-kindness meditation is used to inspire feelings of compassion, kindness, and acceptance toward yourself and others. You open your mind to receive love and then send love to friends, family, and all living beings.

Visualization

Visualization usually starts with a scene, such as a path through the forest coming upon a cool, still lake. In imagining this scene, you're encouraged to incorporate as many senses as possible.

Ho'oponopono

Ho'oponopono is a practice from Native Hawaiians that involves a repeated mantra in which you state the following to a person or even situation that you may be in conflict with:

> *I love you.*
> *I'm sorry.*
> *Please forgive me.*
> *Thank you.*

The "I'm sorry" doesn't mean you are casting blame on yourself. The intent is to release the conflict and your part in it. "Pono" means rightness or completion. This is quite a powerful process. I've often seen people cry when practicing this for the first time. The secret sauce? These words reflect back to the speaker.

Affirmation meditations

Many affirmation meditations are available on YouTube, usually focusing on a specific area, such as wealth, relationships, health, weight loss, anxiety reduction, sleep, releasing anger, or forgiveness. At the end of this book, you'll find affirmations specific to success on your intermittent fasting journey.

CHAPTER 9

The Climacteric Conundrum

As women reach a certain age, the uphill battle we climb with weight loss worsens. Now, instead of trying to scale a concrete mountain wearing roller skates, we do all of that carrying a backpack full of rocks and having developed a mysterious bump across our midlines—leading every woman past the age of 45 to ask, *"What fresh hell is this?"*[55] The fresh hell is perimenopause, menopause, and post-menopause. Collectively, the climacteric.

I'd always prided myself on my small waist. I figured it was the Universe's way of compensating me for the double insult of smallish breasts and thickish thighs. Perimenopause and menopause

---

[55] Heather Corrina authored *What Fresh Hell Is This?: Perimenopause, Menopause, Other Indignities, and You,* Little, Brown Book Group, 2021.

breached our lopsided contract. Like most women experiencing The Change, I was introduced to Belly Fat. Where did this unwelcome visitor come from? And why is its first name always Stubborn?

Turns out, hormones are to blame for this as well. A decrease in estrogen levels leads to an increase in fat across our midsection (belly and hips). Although it's not clear why this happens, fat cells produce estrogen, so one theory is that the body produces more fat cells to compensate for the estrogen loss caused by menopause. *Um ... thanks?*

Why do we need this fickle hormone at all if we're beyond childbearing years? It turns out that estrogen isn't merely a sex and reproductive hormone: It serves many functions in the body, including cognitive, joint, and heart health. So, its loss puts us at a greater risk for many diseases and the damage starts before we exhibit any symptoms. It's natural for our bodies to try to replenish our estrogen levels, but does it have to be with belly fat?!

Dr. Barbie Taylor (known on YouTube as Menopause Taylor) says that when we lose estrogen and don't compensate for its loss, our bodies begin aging. We experience brain loss, our arteries harden, and we increase our risk for osteoporosis, heart disease, and Alzheimer's.[56] When I began exhibiting signs of perimenopause at age 41, a nutritionist friend put it this way: "Early menopause equals early death." *Um ... thanks (again)!*

---

[56] Menopause Q&A with Dr. Barbie Taylor (Menopause Taylor!) https://www.youtube.com/watch?v=vsQJoyn2vxo

Dr. Taylor notes that hormone loss due to perimenopause and menopause occurs in stages, and is a sort of reverse puberty, sending our bodies into chaos. But where puberty turns the hormone switch to "on," the climacteric hits the "off" button.

Then, like the Von Trapp children singing, "So Long, Farewell," from *The Sound of Music*, our hormones begin to leave us in stages. First to go is progesterone, the hormone that supports pregnancy. Its disappearance can leave one feeling wacky, like a geriatric teenager, says Dr. Taylor. Then estrogen packs its bags, which can lead to mood swings, depression, hot flashes, night sweats, and irritability. The form of estrogen that leaves here is estradiol, which I've come to think of as the Divine Feminine of hormones. Estradiol is responsible for maturing and maintaining our reproductive system, the softening of our skin and hair, and (together with testosterone), promoting feelings of sexiness.

Around two years after the departure of estradiol, our testosterone has largely disappeared as well. To compensate for the loss of estradiol, our fat cells produce another type of estrogen called estrone. I think of estrone as estradiol's evil stepsister because, among other goodies, it has been linked to increased cancer risk. [57]

Menopause is uniquely human. Mother Nature, like most TikTokers, assumes we're dead by the time we're 50. The expected

---

[57] Hormone.org "Your Health and Hormones," https://www.hormone.org/your-health-and-hormones/glands-and-hormones-a-to-z/hormones/estrone#:~:text=Specifically%2C%20estrone%20(also%20called%20oestrone,higher%20quantities%20in%20postmenopausal%20women.

Life in Three Acts (Birth, Reproduction, and Death) now has a new act: Life after Reproduction. So, because we're living longer, we also have to live with the consequences of running out of something our bodies depended on for many life-affirming functions. And unless we take steps to compensate for this loss, our health is at risk.

Hormone replacement therapy is an option for some, but not all, and in fact, unless HRT is begun within five to 10 years after the onset of menopause, it's unlikely to do us any good. And the "lucky" ones who sail through menopause with nary a symptom, are unlikely to seek out HRT in the first place. [58]

However, we can take steps to decrease many health risks associated with aging. Let's look at the role intermittent fasting plays.

---

[58] Dr. Taylor believes that many of the health risks associated with HRT are flawed and says that drinking wine carries a similar risk for breast cancer, for instance, but that we "never hear about that." If you decide to try HRT, do your research. Talk to allopathic and naturopathic physicians who specialize in this area.

CHAPTER 10

Anti-Aging and IF

As we age, we lose muscle mass and our metabolism slows, both of which make it harder for us to lose weight. Muscle burns more calories than fat, even at rest. We also lose bone density, making us prone to debilitating injuries. We exercise less, becoming more sedentary. All of this contributes to weight gain and the aging process.

According to the Mayo Clinic, the average woman gains one to two pounds per year during the climacteric period (which can last between five to 10 years). That extra weight can increase our risk for diabetes, cancer, and heart disease.

Regardless of age, insulin is the hormone that has the biggest influence on whether our bodies will store fat. Carbohydrates give our cells fuel when insulin turns carbohydrates into glycogen and delivers it to our cells for energy. But over time, cells can get tired of processing glycogen. When they shut the door to insulin, insulin resistance occurs.

Insulin resistance also increases carb cravings because the cells are no longer taking in the energy they need to function. Because our cells are low on fuel, our bodies think more carbs are the answer and send the message for "More carbs, please!" not yet recognizing that there's plenty of lovely fat to eat. And as Dr. Fung's analogy shows, if we answer that call and feed our bodies carbs from the "fridge," we never tap the fat in the "freezer."

Insulin resistance is also made worse by the increased belly fat that occurs with aging. Yes! Belly fat itself can increase insulin resistance. Per Healthline, "Carrying too much fat around your abdomen promotes inflammation and insulin resistance ... decreasing belly fat leads to increasing insulin sensitivity." [59]Belly fat is made worse by poor sleep and the intake of refined carbs that occurs due to the cravings caused by insulin resistance. Add in a sedentary lifestyle and an increase in the stress hormone, cortisol, and the very natural process of aging becomes the perfect storm for both weight gain, and the inability to shed excess weight. Not to mention increasing our risk for all diseases related to inflammation.

To make weight loss possible and improve our health, we must disrupt this cycle. Intermittent fasting does this by helping us to

---

[59] F. Spritzler, "14 Ways to Lower Your Insulin Levels," Healthline (Sept. 4, 2016) https://www.healthline.com/nutrition

become fat-adapted vs. carb-adapted. It decreases our insulin levels, which decreases our inflammation, reducing our risk for inflammation-related diseases, and it also combats many of the effects of aging. I love to watch YouTube videos of weight loss transformation and read articles with before and after photos of significant weight loss. And you know what? In almost every case, the image in the *after* photo looks like they could be the *before* person's daughter or son. Losing weight takes years off a person's appearance. There is an old wives' tale you may have heard, "After a certain age, you can either have your face or your ass." Some people believe that when we lose weight after a certain age, it can make our faces look older, gaunt, and make wrinkles more pronounced (the opposite of plumping up with Botox or Juvederm). But it's a rare "after" photo that doesn't also look like a decade or so had disappeared along with the extra weight. Speaking strictly for myself, I know I look younger when I'm slimmer.

But beyond weight loss and a youthful appearance, intermittent fasting can reverse many of the effects of aging. Don't believe me? Let's hear it from Luke Corey, a registered dietitian with the Mayo Clinic Sports Medicine: "Fasting … slows down the degradation of DNA, which is what occurs when we age, and accelerates DNA repair, thus slowing down the aging process."

Fasting also increases the levels of antioxidants that can help prevent the body's cells from being broken down by free radicals, which are molecules that can cause damage to cells. Additionally, fasting can reduce the chronic inflammation that occurs as people age. Intermittent fasting can help us live a better quality of life for a longer period of time. What's not to love about that?

A study at the Okinawa Institute of Science and Technology Graduate University found that fasting not only increases metabolism, "it may also reverse the aging process." The study showed that it is the metabolic changes that occur during fasting that lead to its rejuvenating effects.[60]

---

[60] "New Evidence Shows Fasting May Slow Down Aging," Being Patient, (Feb. 1, 2019)

CHAPTER 11

Fast Drivers

PICTURE YOURSELF IN YOUR FAVORITE VACATION SPOT or perhaps somewhere you've always wanted to go. You're laughing, talking with friends, and having the time of your life. Which "you" did you bring to this idyll? Are you feeling healthy and vibrant and full of life, able to keep up with the group? Or are you retiring early, passing on active adventures, cringing when a camera is aimed in your direction?

Do you feel great, proud, vibrantly alive?

Setting aside my tongue-in-cheek references to wanting a body like Jennifer Aniston's, comparing our bodies to others', particularly those of celebrities, isn't healthy. In an episode of *Roseanne*, her TV daughter asked, "Mom, what's anorexia?" Roseanne answered, "Oh, that's a disease women get from reading too many magazines."

That's not far from the truth. Food is our friend. Try not to think of food as "good food" or "bad food." There are some toxic non-food substances out there, and you should avoid them as much as possible. But if 80-90% of your food intake promotes your good health and you're feeling good energy, enjoy your food and love your life.

A healthy, well-lived life should be your ultimate goal. That said, there's nothing wrong with wanting to be the hottest version of you. What is your fasting driver? You will likely need to keep it in mind when the going gets tough. And fasting, especially when you first try it, can be tough. It can call on inner resources and make you dig deep. But the more you do it, the easier it becomes. Like a lot of life skills, success at fasting is mostly mental, and success is cumulative.

Fast Driver 1: I'd Like to Be the Weight on My Driver's License

Why do some jurisdictions require you to put your weight on your driver's license? Is the police officer who pulls you over really going to know the difference?

Intermittent fasting can help you achieve your weight loss goals. That is something no diet can honestly say, with the possible exception of going 100% keto, which I find to be unsustainable. If you want to fit into a size 12, or 6, or 2, you can do it with intermittent fasting. You should aim for a healthy weight, however.

I recently responded to a Facebook post from a woman on a fasting group I belong to who was aiming for a weight of 150 lbs.: *I'm almost 5'4 but I wear a size 8, so even though I should be in the 130s, I think that's too low for my body type.*

I congratulated her for knowing her own body and not taking weight charts as gospel.

So, the following are guidelines—but only guidelines—to determine a healthy weight range. Variables in human body, shape, and composition reduce their reliability. In short, I like to say that there are lies, damned lies, and weight charts.

Body mass index

According to the Center for Disease Control, we should all aim for a body mass index (BMI) of between 18.5 and 24.9. [61] Here's the breakdown:

- If your BMI is less than 18.5, it falls within the underweight range.
- If your BMI is 18.5 to 24.9, it falls within the normal or healthy weight range.
- If your BMI is 25.0 to 29.9, it falls within the overweight range.
- If your BMI is 30.0 or higher, it falls within the obese range.

---

[61] "Assessing Your Weight," CDC (May 25, 2021) https://www.cdc.gov/healthyweight/assessing/index.html#:~:text=If%20your%20BMI%20is%2018.5,falls%20within%20the%20obese%20range

Says the chart. To determine your BMI, take your weight in kilograms and divide it by the square of your height in meters. There are BMI calculators available on the web that can convert from the metric system and run the calculations for you. Here's an example: A person weighing 160 pounds who is 5′7″ tall would have a BMI of 25.1, which, by this chart edges just into the "overweight" category.

Waist measurement

The CDC also has a guideline for waist measurement. Too much abdominal fat (hello, bread belly, I'm talkin' to you) can place us at a higher risk for obesity-related conditions, such as type 2 diabetes, high blood pressure, and coronary heart disease. This risk is greater for these individuals:

- Men with a waist measurement greater than 40 inches
- Women (unless pregnant) with a waist measurement greater than 35 inches

Waist-to-hip ratio

Medical News Today offers other ways to determine appropriate weight and shape. One of these is the waist-to-hip ratio.[62]

To determine yours, first measure around the narrowest part of your waist. Next, divide this measurement by the widest part of your hips. For instance, for a 31″-waist measurement and a 40″-hip measurement, you would divide 31 by 40, which is .775 (rounded to .78). This is an indicator of cardiovascular health.

---

[62] Yvette Brazier, "How much should I weigh for my height and age?" *Medical News Today* (Jan 18, 2020)
https://www.medicalnewstoday.com/articles/323446#waist-hip-ratio

In males:

- A ratio below 0.9 indicates low risk.
- A ratio from 0.8 to 0.89 indicates moderate risk.
- A ratio of 0.9 and above indicate high risk.

In females:

- A ratio below 0.8 indicates low risk.
- A ratio from 0.8 to 0.89 indicates moderate risk.
- A ratio of 0.9 and above indicates high risk.

Body fat percentage

Body fat percentage is the weight of a person's fat divided by their total weight.

The optimal body fat percentage varies by activity level. Acceptable ranges for people with average activity levels are 18–25% for males and 25–31% for females.

To measure body fat percentage, there are several options. With skin caliper tests, a health professional measures the fat tissue on your thigh, abdomen, chest (for men) or upper arm (for women). Hydrostatic body fat testing is underwater weighing. Other high-tech options include air densitometry (which measures air displacement), dual energy X-ray absorptiometry, and bioelectrical impedance analysis. (Say those three times fast.)

As *Medical News Today* reports, *none* of these give a completely accurate reading, and each is at best a reasonable assessment.

Waist-to-Height Ratio

If you haven't had enough number crunching, here's another one: the waist-to-height ratio. As you may suspect, this involves dividing your waist measurement by your height in inches. Anything less than 50% is in the healthy range. Anything over 50%—not so much. Following are figures provided by healthline.com:

Waist to Height Ratio	Underweight	Healthy Weight	Overweight	Obese
Females	Less than 42%	42–48%	49–57%	Greater than 58%
Males	Less than 43%	43–52%	53–62%	Greater than 63%

Big-boned?

Don't obsess over these numbers. There are plenty of reasons why these measurements don't work for some people. Some people are just built differently, and waist and hip measurements will fall outside the norm no matter what. There's also the argument that some people are just "big-boned." A practical test with doubtful scientific merit is to wrap one hand around the opposite wrist with your thumb and middle finger touching. If they just meet, you have an average frame. If they overlap, you have a small frame. If they fail to meet, you have a large frame and can proudly wear the "I'm Just Big-Boned" sweatshirt. (If there was one, and there probably is.)

Fitness level

Weight is only one indicator of fitness. The Mayo Clinic measures fitness in several ways. For instance, a fit person:

- Has a resting heart rate of 60–100 beats per minute
- Should be able to run 1.5 miles in 11–14 minutes for males, 13–17.5 minutes for females.

The above running time depends on age. For women, this breaks down as follows:

- Age 25: 13 minutes
- Age 35: 13.5 minutes
- Age 45: 14 minutes
- Age 55: 16 minutes
- Age 65: 17.5 minutes

A fit woman should also be able to do the following number of pushups without needing to stop to rest:

- Age 25: 20 pushups
- Age 35: 19 pushups
- Age 45: 14 pushups
- Age 55: 10 pushups
- Age 65: 10 pushups

Given that the Mayo Clinic requires you to lower your body with each pushup until your chin touches the floor, I'm currently in great shape for a 125-year-old.

The sit-up test

The sit-up test measures the strength and endurance of your abdominal muscles. Lie on the floor with your knees bent at a 90-degree angle, feet flat on the floor. Cross your arms across your chest and raise your head and shoulders off the floor, leaving your sit-upon where it is. Then return to the down position. Do as many as you can in one minute. For a good fitness level, women should strive for these numbers:

- Age 25: 39 sit-ups
- Age 35: 30 sit-ups
- Age 45: 25 sit-ups
- Age 55: 21 sit-ups
- Age 65: 12 sit-ups

Shockingly, given that my abdominal muscles are weak, and I hate crunches, I was able to do more than 50 of these. If I had to sit up more than merely lifting my head and shoulders off the floor, that number would have been drastically reduced.

Flexibility

The Mayo Clinic also offers a sit-and-reach test to determine the flexibility of your legs, hips, and lower back. Secure a yardstick on the floor, with tape at the 15-inch mark. Sit on the floor, placing the soles of your feet even with that mark. Slowly reach forward as far as you can, exhaling and holding the position for at least one second.

Note the distance of your reach. Repeat this test twice more and record the best of three. "Good" flexibility for women follows:

- Age 25: 21.5 inches
- Age 35: 20.5 inches
- Age 45: 20 inches
- Age 55: 19 inches
- Age 65: 17.5 inches

The Mayo Clinic advises you to repeat these tests every six weeks as you strive to improve your results.

Fast Driver 2: I'd Like to Keep Both of My Feet, Thank You

According to the CDC, more than one in three American adults has prediabetes, and 84% of those don't know they have it. Prediabetes increases the risk of developing type 2 diabetes, heart disease, and stroke.[63] Risk factors for prediabetes per the CDC include:

- Being overweight
- Being 45 or older
- Having a parent, brother, or sister with type 2 diabetes
- Being physically active fewer than three times per week
- Having gestational diabetes or giving birth to a baby who weighed more than 9 pounds

---

[63] "Prediabetes - Your Chance to Prevent Type 2 Diabetes," CDC.gov (May 25, 2021) https://www.cdc.gov/diabetes/basics/prediabetes.html

- Having polycystic ovary syndrome

Perhaps you have a family history of health issues such as obesity, type 2 diabetes, or other health concerns, and you'd rather history not repeat itself. Or you may want to set a good example for the next generation. As we've learned, intermittent fasting is a great way to take control of your health, prevent many common health maladies— including many types of cancer—and reverse symptoms of the following:

- Obesity
- High blood pressure
- Type 2 diabetes and prediabetes

The American Diabetes Association (ADA) recommends that most adults begin screening for diabetes at age 45, or sooner if they're overweight or have additional risk factors.

There are several blood tests for prediabetes. Three follow.

Glycated hemoglobin (A1C) test

This test shows your average blood sugar level for the past three months. It measures the percentage of blood sugar attached to the oxygen-carrying protein in your red blood cells (hemoglobin). Higher blood sugar levels equate to more hemoglobin with sugar attached. Per the ADA:

- An A1C level below 5.7% is considered normal

- An A1C level between 5.7% and 6.4% is considered prediabetes
- An A1C level of 6.5% or higher on two separate tests indicates type 2 diabetes

Fasting blood sugar test

With this test, a blood sample is taken after you fast for at least eight hours or overnight.

- A fasting blood sugar level below 100 milligrams per deciliter (mg/dL)—5.6 millimoles per liter (mmol/L)—is considered normal.
- A fasting blood sugar level from 100 to 125 mg/dL (5.6 to 7.0 mmol/L) is considered prediabetes. This result is sometimes called impaired fasting glucose.
- A fasting blood sugar level at or above 126 mg/dL (7.0 mmol/L) indicates type 2 diabetes.

Oral glucose tolerance test

This test is usually used to diagnose diabetes during pregnancy. First, you fast for at least eight hours, then you drink a sugary solution, and your blood sugar level will be measured again after two hours. When I was pregnant with our first son, this test caused me to have such a sugar crash that I was an emotional wreck for hours. (Apparently, I failed the glucose tolerance test.)

I phoned my birthing coach, sobbing, and she insisted I hang up and make myself a peanut butter sandwich immediately. Maybe she just wanted to get hysterical me off the phone, but it worked. I made a peanut butter sandwich, and in just a few moments, I began to feel normal again. (I refused this test with my second pregnancy.)

- With this test, a blood sugar level less than 140 mg/dL (7.8 mmol/L) is considered normal.
- A blood sugar level from 140 to 199 mg/dL (7.8 to 11.0 mmol/L) is considered prediabetes. This level is sometimes referred to as impaired glucose tolerance.
- A blood sugar level at or above 200 mg/dL (11.1 mmol/L) indicates type 2 diabetes.

If you have prediabetes, take steps to reverse it (intermittent fasting is one solution, low carb is another) and have your blood sugar levels checked at least once per year. If you have type 2 diabetes, ask your doctor about intermittent fasting and carb reduction to improve your symptoms.

The ADA recommends several steps to limit risk. I would consider them in addition to, and not in lieu of, intermittent fasting, given its success rate for obesity and type 2 diabetes:

- **Eat healthy.** Eat a variety of foods to help you achieve your goals without compromising taste or nutrition.
- **Be more active.** Aim for at least 150 minutes of moderate or 75 minutes of vigorous aerobic activity each week.

- **Lose excess weight.** Losing just 5% to 7% of your body weight—about 14 pounds (6.4 kilograms) if you weigh 200 pounds (91 kilograms)—can reduce your risk for type 2 diabetes. Focus on permanent changes to your eating and exercise habits.
- **Stop smoking.** Smoking can lead to weight loss. You probably didn't expect to hear that, but it's true. It can increase metabolic rate and decrease caloric absorption, reducing appetite.[64] And yet, according to the CDC, it is the leading cause of preventable death in the United States, causing more than 480,000 deaths per year. Per the CDC, "More than 10 times as many US citizens have died prematurely from smoking than died in all the wars fought by the United States." Outside of illegal drug use, being a smoker likely has a bigger negative effect on our health than anything else we voluntarily do.

Secondhand smoke is also a risk factor. I go to great lengths to avoid secondhand smoke because it makes my eyes sting and water and my throat constrict. I can't fathom how some people think it's acceptable to breathe out a carcinogen around others, especially around babies and children. If I'm walking down a sidewalk and see

---

[64] Arnaud Chiolero et al, "Consequences of smoking for body weight, body fat distribution, and insulin resistance," *The American Journal of Clinical Nutrition*, Volume 87, Issue 4 (April 2008), pages 801-809
https://academic.oup.com/ajcn/article/87/4/801/4633357

someone ahead of me who's smoking, I'll either hang way back or cross the street to avoid them.

Although primarily linked to lung cancer, smoking can cause cancer anywhere in the body. It can result in preterm delivery for pregnant women, stillbirth, low birth weight, ectopic pregnancy, and facial clefts in infants.

Women who smoke have weaker bones than women who have never smoked and therefore have an increased risk of broken bones. It can also affect the health of teeth and gums and cause tooth loss. It can increase risk of cataracts and make type 2 diabetes harder to control (and it increases the risk of developing diabetes in the first place by 30–40%). It can increase inflammation and decrease immune function. And it can cause rheumatoid arthritis.

And it hasn't looked cool since James Dean did it in *Rebel Without a Cause* in 1955.

Fast Driver 3: The Ponce de Leon Effect

Wrinkle cream buyers notwithstanding, the person most associated with the search for the fountain of youth is the 16th-century Spanish explorer, Juan Ponce de Leon. If only he'd known about IF!

As we've seen, beneficial changes occur at the cellular level when your body is in a fasting state, whether the fast is temporary or intermittent. Several of these changes work together to promote a longer, healthier life. Per BioAge Health, these changes include:

- Cellular repair. Cells remove wastes that would cause cellular damage, which can lead to aging.
- Gene expression. Changes occur in genes that promote longevity and prevent disease.
- Hormones. A drop in insulin levels helps prevent diabetes and may boost longevity.
- Inflammation reduction. Inflammation is associated with many diseases.
- Oxidative stress protection. This prevents cell damage due to unstable molecules, called free radicals.

Intermittent fasting also helps you lose weight and abdominal fat, which in turn improves your health and prevents chronic diseases that can shorten your life.[65]

The antiaging benefits are the number-one reason I choose to do IF. It's not out of vanity (well, not *mostly*) but out of a desire to be there for my sons. I'd like to extend my life (and health) as long as possible.

Two books to check out, if antiaging is your Big Why, are *Younger Next Year: Live Strong, Fit, and Sexy Until You're 80 and Beyond,* by Chris Crowley and Henry S. Lodge, and Linus Pauling's *How to Live Longer and Feel Better.*

---

[65] "How Intermittent Fasting Can Help to Fight Aging," *BioAge Health* (May 25, 2021) https://www.bioagehealth.com/how-intermittent-fasting-can-help-to-fight-aging/

Younger Next Year calls out our "sedentary, all-feast, no-famine culture" as a reason we age in poor health—something intermittent fasting can solve.

Pauling is a molecular chemist who won a Nobel Prize for his chemistry work and another one for peace. His book, *How to Live Longer and Feel Better,* which he wrote at age 85, touts the use of mega doses of vitamin C, exercise, and reducing sugar and alcohol.

Obviously, there's living longer, and then there's living healthier for longer, and these are not the same thing. Aim for living as healthy a life as possible, and the antiaging benefits will follow.

Fast Driver 4: Optimal Health

Optimal health doesn't simply mean free of disease. It means fit, vibrant, and fully alive.

To gain optimal health, **avoid putting toxins into your body**. cigarettes, misuse of alcohol and drugs, processed and prepackaged foods, and foods that contain pesticides, growth hormones, and mercury, among other toxins. Avoid using toxic household cleaners and weed killers, and avoid being around toxins in the work environment. Avoid sugar as much as possible, using it for a rare treat if at all, and avoid trans fats, often found in packaged baked goods.

Instead, **eat nourishing foods**, as close to nature as possible, and eat a variety of fruits and vegetables (heavy on the vegetables).

Get exercise, including weight-bearing exercise. Using your muscles is extremely important for optimal health. Lifting weights lowers blood sugar and insulin levels, improves cholesterol levels, and lowers triglycerides. It also raises levels of testosterone (yes, we need it too, ladies) and growth hormones—both important to optimal health. Exercise can also help prevent depression and reduce the risk of obesity, type 2 diabetes, Alzheimer's, and other diseases; plus, it can help reduce fat.

Sleep well. We covered the importance of sleep and exercise earlier. Sleep has a lot of the same benefits as exercise. There is nothing brave, noble, or admirable about foregoing sleep to power through a work project. I used to be proud of being able to pull an all-nighter for work until I read *Why We Sleep*, by Dr. Matthew Walker, PhD, and learned that not only was I not doing my body any favors, but I was also actually doing irreparable harm. There is no "catching up on sleep" from a biological standpoint. One night's missed sleep and too little sleep, particularly the right kind of sleep, has permanent consequences. Aim for a minimum of seven hours, and preferably eight, and your body and your health will thank you.

Avoid excess stress. While some stress is good for us (called eustress), excess stress can raise our cortisol levels, impair our metabolism, increase food cravings, add to belly fat stores, and raise our risk of disease and depression. Ways to relieve stress include exercise, getting out in nature, meditation, and deep breathing techniques.

Get appropriate health screenings. In addition to the recommended diabetes screening at age 45, the new age to screen for colorectal cancer and get your first colonoscopy is also 45. This is due to younger people being diagnosed with advanced colon cancer far earlier than the previously recommended screening age of 50. When I had a recent colonoscopy (my third, due to family history), I asked the doctor why people were being diagnosed with advanced colorectal cancer at such young ages. She said, "I don't know, but I suspect it's diet." If you have a family history of colon cancer, like me, you should also consider screening earlier than age 45.

CHAPTER 12

Food Dreams and Flashcards: My 14-Day Fast

OTHER THAN MY COUSIN, who lost 100 pounds on keto (combined with occasional intermittent fasting), at first, I didn't tell anyone I had decided to do a 14-day fast—not even the people who know that I occasionally do fasts of three to five days. I knew it would be a challenge for me, and I didn't need anyone fueling my doubt with their well-intentioned concern.

So, how did it go? Following are journal entries from my fast, with a few comments to you, dear goddess.

Day 1: Starting weight: 144 lbs. My weight was technically within the "normal" range for my height (5´5″), but I felt bloated, and my muffin top looked more like rising bread dough that overflowed the mixing bowl. Because my jeans were a tight fit, I mostly wore yoga pants or pajama bottoms during the day unless I had to go somewhere, in which case I suffered the squeeze.

Because I'm "fat adapted" due to being a frequent intermittent faster, I wasn't hungry at all the first day, but it was a very busy day, and I didn't go to bed until almost 2 a.m. Then I couldn't sleep. I got up and worked a bit, then went back to bed again around 3:30 a.m., when I did finally sleep, but my day started again at 6:30 a.m. So, I got about 2 ½ hours of sleep. Not a good start.

Day 2: Weight: 142.8 lbs. A loss of 1.2 pounds! This was a key day. I had my first doctor's appointment in years (to get a referral for a colonoscopy). While there, I got a blood test for lipids, thyroid, cholesterol, and blood sugar levels. I was cold and dressed in layers, but temps were in the 40s, so that's to be expected. Again, I wasn't hungry, but I was tempted to eat some leftover roast chicken while preparing my son's chicken quesadillas. However, it was fairly easy to avoid eating. Around 3 p.m., I started to get super tired (from lack of sleep the night before), but I had plenty to do, so I was able to keep busy until 9:30, when I took a multivitamin plus potassium, went to bed, and slept well.

Day 3: Weight: 141 lbs. A loss of 1.8 pounds, three pounds overall. After I weighed, I checked for results in my full-length bathroom mirror. My stomach was definitely flatter.

I felt good all day. I didn't feel any true hunger, but I did feel like eating a few times. When that happened, I drank water or took a bit of Himalayan salt and the feeling passed. It's amazing how a bit of salt helps. It also helps to stay busy, and I did—working on this book, playing with my dog, and responding to emails, phone calls, and Facebook posts. I've done multiple three-day fasts before, so this was familiar territory for me. I've also done a five-day fast, so I know that the next two days are doable. It will take untapped strength to get through Days 6–14 but knowing that I have you to report back to helps. So, thank you!

Day 4: Weight: 139.4 lbs. I woke at 4:40 a.m. (after waking several times during the night). I stayed in bed until 6 a.m. and realized I was thirsty. I had a glass of water on my nightstand, but I wanted to weigh empty, so I waited. I should report now that I've done zero exercise during this time. I've been working on the book, researching, basically all day and much of the night. So, these losses are from fasting only.

I will start taking some bone broth if I feel I need it. Pretty good energy all day and not hungry at all.

Day 5: Weight: 137.8 lbs. That's another 1.6 pounds gone! Did not sleep well. Woke at 2 a.m. feeling like I was done with sleep. I took another melatonin (my third of the night), but it wasn't working. I think my body is energized from all the fat it's consuming. I felt draggy today, so I took ¾ cup of bone broth with plenty of black pepper. It. Was. Delicious.

Day 6: Weight: 136 lbs. That's another 1.8 pounds (!) shed at a point where I thought my weight loss would surely be slowing down. I think my body is saying, "Thank you for shedding this fat I've been carrying around; lemme help." We'll see what the next eight days bring. Slept well last night. I'm in uncharted territory now; I've never fasted for this long.

I had great energy all day and wasn't hungry. Well, there were a couple of moments. My son needed help with his culinary arts flashcards, and I had to read descriptions like "Which international cuisine is known for thick wheat yeast bread seasoned with coriander, ginger, honey, orange peel, and cinnamon?" Later, when I was making him High Nachos, I was only tempted by the tortilla chips (my weakness and a definite trigger food), but I quickly closed the bag and started doing the dishes to distract myself. It worked. Later, I rewarded this display of virtue with a cup of bone broth. Again, superb. And although my stomach is still in bread dough territory, I'm beginning to look less matronly in my jeans. Woot woot.

Day 7: Weight: 136 lbs. First day of no weight loss. I expected this at some point. To be honest, the huge drops I saw on Days 3–6 (mostly water weight loss, I'm sure) were surprising. I consider a little plateauing part of the process. I slept well last night but woke at 4:30 a.m., and that was it for sleeping, so I only had about six hours of sleep. Today I really needed to tap my inner strength. Not that I was hungry, just that food was starting to sound *really good.* I wanted to eat my arm. And once again, my son needed help with his culinary arts flash cards. Luckily, I had already heated up some bone broth, which I sipped while reading out definitions for *confit*, *rémoulade*, and fish *en papillote*. (Beef broth is not only tasty but also helps preserve one's arm.)

A funny thing happened today: I was making an appointment for my colonoscopy, and the intake scheduler asked me a bunch of medical questions. Then she got to "And what is your weight?" I didn't know how to answer that question. I finally said, "That depends. What date will I be coming in?" We settled on a date, and I made up a number and told her I'd call her if anything changed.

Day 8: Weight: 136 lbs. (yes, still). This is what's known as a temporary plateau, goddess. It will happen. And if weight loss were the only benefit to fasting, I'd be incredibly disappointed, natch. But I'm in this for other reasons, and I'm in it for the duration. It's possible, too, that I've not been drinking quite enough water, which I'll remedy today.

I had what's left of the bone broth (3/4 cup) at 11 a.m., followed by coffee with one tablespoon (I measured) of half and half. Half and half is NOT fasting friendly (if you need to add cream, use full-fat cream, which contains no carbs), but I'm beginning to feel a little like Oliver Twist. And half and half only has 0.5 grams of carbs, 20 calories. If I gain weight from that, I'm going to ask to be put in a medically induced coma until I start losing again. Not that I'm bitter.

Day 9: Weight: 134.8 lbs. Hold the pentobarbital! I have good energy—better than the last couple of days. In fact, it feels like my cells are *singing*. Am I losing my mind? I slept for about four hours initially, but after getting up at 5 a.m. and dealing with some email, I went back to sleep until after 7 a.m.

In other news, I'm beginning to think that hot baths on an extended fast are not a good idea. My go-to way to relax (besides a glass of red, currently verboten) is a hot bath with Epsom salts. But there's something about the change in body temperature when I got out that made me feel like I was falling off a cliff. So, I sat on a towel on the bathroom floor for about 20 minutes until that feeling passed.

No bone broth today (it was homemade, and I ran out), but overall, it was a good day.

Day 10: Weight: 134.6 lbs. Had a good night's sleep. Woke at 6:30 a.m. feeling fantastic. More singing from the cell choir. And BIG news: I'm almost positive that a 22-year-old shoulder injury has resolved itself! I only hope that the foot injury caused by those use-more-muscle-when-you-walk "fitness" shoes has also resolved—that would be a game changer! That injury only flares up when I overdo it, though, and I'm not about to test it during this fast.

I mowed my front and back lawn today, taking a couple of water breaks because I tired more easily than usual. Later, I went clothes shopping but came back empty-handed. Sadly, I don't have Jennifer Aniston's body yet.

I had to really draw on my inner strength today. Even though I only have a full four days left, I miss food. I miss the mouth taste, the chewing, the swallowing, the feeling of something—anything—in my stomach. I just keep coming back to my goals and the fact that I'll have to report back to you on my progress. That keeps me between the bumpers.

Day 11: Weight: 134.4 lbs. At some point, seeing the numbers drop, I thought, "Wouldn't it be amazing if I could make it to 130 (a drop of 14 pounds) in 14 days?" It doesn't look like that's going to happen now, losing just 0.2 pounds each day over the past two days, but I'm not complaining.

I had a minor setback today. I had to pick up some medicine for my son at the pharmacy and phoned him on the way back to see if he'd like a donut as a treat. Of course, he said yes. I stopped by Sesame Donut and ordered two of his favorites (willpower that he has, he's saving one for tomorrow), and got myself a large coffee while I was there. I wasn't even tempted by the donuts. The clerk asked, "Would you like cream in that?"

I should have said no, but I answered, "Sure, let's walk on the wild side." He was training a new recruit, showing her the ropes, and swirled a bunch of cream—far more than I would have even on a non-fasting day—before I could say, "That's enough!" I swear there had to be at least ¼ cup of cream in there. I should have asked for a different mix or poured it out when I got home, but instead, I just used it to doctor my own coffee over the rest of the morning.

Today I'm feeling ... well, maybe a story would help. When I was first dating the man who would become my husband and the father of my children, he offered to train me to run. He belonged to a running group, had completed 20 marathons, and thought running would be something fun we could do together. I was a willing novice. We trained for a few weeks, and at one point, he told me I was ready for my first double-digit run. I was nervous, but we chose Forest Park in Portland, Oregon, which has some beautiful running trails, and I was hoping the scenery would distract me from what I was about to ask my body to do—10 miles of jogging.

Unfortunately, it had rained the day before, and the trails were mucky. This made running treacherous, and I had to watch every step rather than enjoy my surroundings. On top of this, the muck coated my running shoes, adding additional weight to my stride. It was hard, but I dug down, persevered, and sooner than I thought possible, my boyfriend slash running coach said, "We're almost there. It's just around the next bend." Thinking we'd only done about seven miles, I was thrilled that we'd already done 10! I couldn't wait to reach "there"! But when we got "there," he said, "This is the halfway point; now we turn around and go back."

My body had already let down, and I couldn't imagine completing another five miles. I cursed him silently, then audibly, for not being clear in his communication. I felt set up, frankly. He offered to call it quits for the day and walk back together, but I was too angry (and if I'm being honest, too stubborn) to let the situation keep me from achieving what I set out to do. I turned around and began running, feeling hot tears stream down my face; feeling my feet, heavy with mud, slipping and sliding; feeling the ache in my legs and back, the lump in my throat, and the fire in my lungs. I ran that last five miles half blind and more than half steamed.

All that is to say: I'm at the "there" point in this 14-day fast, even though I only have four days left. It's become very hard. I'd really like to eat something! But I'm no less stubborn today than I was all those years ago. I know this is good for me, and I intend to achieve what I set out to do. So, I'll push on, even though I have no anger to fuel me for this leg of the journey. But at least there's no muck.

I had another cup of bone broth today. I like the brand called Kettle & Fire, which is made from grass-fed beef. Look for the highest quality bone broth (or make your own, as I usually do). I'll put an easy recipe in the back of this book. It couldn't be simpler.

Day 12: Weight: 134 lbs. Every day now feels like climbing a mountain. Self-care is the Sherpa. I had some bone broth, took a warm (not hot) bath, rested as much as possible, got and took the correct magnesium formula (Whole Foods only had 99 mg potassium, and I'm not taking 10 capsules to get to the recommended 1,000 mg dosage).

For some reason, coffee didn't taste good today, even with a splash of half-and-half. I poured it out.

I made my son Shoyu Chicken for dinner, and the smell of garlic, ginger, and coconut aminos drove me wild. He naturally had it over a huge pile of white rice (he can eat carbs and not gain an ounce, but I love him anyway). When he got up midway through his meal to get something just as I was walking past, I fantasized about burying my face in his plate, Rottweiler style.

Two. Days. To. Go.

Day 13: Weight: 133 lbs. I'm surprised at the one-pound drop this late in the fast, and I'm thinking it might be that I'm a little dehydrated. I drank a good amount of water yesterday, but maybe I was a little shy of the right amount. I think the new magnesium formula helped because last night I had the best night of sleep since the fast began. At breakfast I had a nice espresso with a splash of half-and-half, and it was delicious.

Win! I was able to comfortably wear a pair of jeans that has been sitting on the top shelf of my closet for two years!

Day 14: Weight: 134.2 lbs. A *gain* of 1.2 pounds? Odd. Maybe it was dehydration yesterday, and now I'm plumped back up. I didn't overdo water by any stretch of the imagination, though. I have a highly accurate digital scale, but it does require a level surface. I tried moving it around and weighing again: same results. This sort of sucks, but, in a way, I'm glad it happened because it can happen when you do an extended fast, and it doesn't take away from the many benefits of fasting. It's just a temporary number on a scale, so don't give it any more power than that. Also, it's best not to weigh every day, as I have been. I'm only doing it so I can report to you.

I had an okay night sleeping last night. Woke at 3 a.m. and had to take a second melatonin but was able to get back to sleep. I had another food dream. In this one, I ate two pieces of homemade chocolate fudge. I could feel myself eating it, tasting the butter I'd used to coat the pan, the weighty sweetness of the fudge on my tongue. Then in my dream I thought, "It's Day 14! I blew it!" At that, I woke up and realized it was only a dream.

I feel great today! Not because it's the last day (well, maybe some of that) but because I feel as though I could go on longer if I wanted to (*I don't wanna, and you can't make me*). Yesterday was also fairly easy. I had been pushing myself too hard on a work project and decided to back way off, watched an old movie in the evening instead of working. Fasting is hard enough. You need to be kind to yourself in other areas. Despite backing off a lot, it was still a busy day.

Day 15: Fasting is Done! Final Weight: 134.2 lbs. I woke at 3 a.m. and didn't get back to sleep again even after taking a melatonin. So much for the new magnesium formula being the perfect cure. I have a strong desire for an omelet with green onions, but reintroducing food carefully is important. Today will be fermented foods, bone broth, and steamed veggies. Yay! I get to chew (a little). But before I eat anything, I've scheduled a follow-up blood test. I offered to do private pay, but my doctor wouldn't order a repeated blood test so soon after the first one. "Not much will change," she said. So, I made an appointment with an independent lab.

Results After 14-Day Fast

Marker	Standard Range	Fasted (Day 2)	Fasted (Day 15)
Weight	117-144 (5'5" female)	144	134.2
Cholesterol	Less than/equal to 199	242	212
HDL	Greater than/equal to 40	66	58
LDL	Less than/equal to 99	158	140
Triglycerides	Less than/equal to 149	89	78
Glucose	Less than/equal to 99 prediabetes: 100-125 Diabetes: greater than or equal to 126	105	81
Average glucose over 30 days (estimated)	Same as above	114	103

Summary of the fast

My glucose level went from a prediabetes level to well within normal for the single-day test. The 30-day test also improved, but since it's an estimate, I'm not too worried about that extra 5 or 6 points in prediabetes territory (though it's something to watch).

My triglycerides dropped, my LDL dropped, and my HDL also dropped (that one isn't so good, but it's still at a very good number).

My cholesterol is still a bit high (but it dropped 30 points). I'm also not worried about cholesterol because I don't follow the Standard American Diet (SAD) and I do allow plenty of healthy fats into my diet.

Overall, I'm very happy with these results. I met with my doctor after the second labs were in. She was curious about the changes but told me she had no concerns about my initial labs, feeling they were well within the healthy range for my age. Also, I was tested on Day 2 of my fast. My improvements may have been even more impressive had I had the initial blood work done a couple of days earlier.

So, would I do another 14-day fast? I'm not sure. Days 11 and 12 were ridiculously hard. As I write this, though, I'm in the middle of a 10-day fast. I want to see if those singing cells have learned any new tunes.

CHAPTER 13

Goddess in the Kitchen: Recipes and Pantry Items

THIS IS A GUIDE, NOT A COOKBOOK, and I'm not a gourmet chef. I tend to find a few staples I make over and over, occasionally adding new recipes I run across that sound yummy and doable. If they're a hit and straightforward to make, they get added to the rotation. I'm only including the few recipes I specifically mentioned in this book (plus a few others that you may find helpful), and I trust you to know, find, or be able to invent better ones. With the last recipe, I've mentioned a couple of cookbooks I like, where you may find some new staples of your own. I've also included some nice-to-have items for the pantry.

Recipes

Bone broth

Bone broth is so good for you, especially when fasting or breaking a fast. Not only does it contain collagen, but it also contains the all-important potassium and magnesium, plus proline, glycine, calcium, and phosphorous, among other goodies. As such, it's good for hair, skin, nails, connective tissues, bones, and ligaments. It also has gut-healing nutrients, very important during and after a fast. You can buy it in health stores in liquid or powdered form, but making your own is a cinch.

I usually make chicken bone broth because we don't eat a lot of red meat, and when we do, it's usually ground. We do, however, make a lot of roasted chicken. You make chicken bone broth by placing the carcass, skin, and bones of a roasted chicken into a crockpot. Then add water or chicken broth, veggies (onions and celery are good choices), pepper, and salt, and leave it to simmer on low overnight. In the morning, strain it into freezer-safe containers, keeping enough for your immediate needs in the refrigerator. I usually pick through the bones for meat, as well, and use it to make chicken soup, add it to a salad, or make chicken quesadillas. A budget saver!

Beef bone broth is similarly made, using bones from beef. You can sometimes talk your favorite grocer into giving or selling you a bag o' bones. Be sure to get bones from grass-fed (and, if possible, grass-finished) beef because it's the richest in nutrients.

Fish bone broth is also possible and just as nutritious, and for those who prefer not to eat land animals, it's a great option. I did learn, however, that you should use non-oily fish, so the oil doesn't turn rancid during simmering. Try halibut, cod, sole, rockfish, or turbot. Avoid farm-raised Frankenfish. Start with 5–7 pounds of fish bones, carcasses, or heads, add spices, herbs, and vegetables to taste, and simmer as above.

What about that layer of fat? When bone broth cools, the fat separates from the broth. It's up to you whether you want to remove or keep this, but a keto enthusiast would say, "That's the best part!" and would consider it sacrilege to skim it off. I never remove the fat for two reasons: Fat is good for us, and it makes the broth thicker.

"Bone broth" for vegans

Although I'm not a huge meat eater, I do eat meat, and I don't want to leave our vegan friends out of the equation. I found a delicious-sounding recipe for Gut-Healing Vegetable Broth on wallflowerkitchen.com and have noted its URL below.[66]

Veggie frittata

This is one of my go-to options to get veggies into a breakfast-type meal—*breakfast-type* because I tend to postpone eating until at least 10:30 or 11 a.m., a time of eating which most people would call brunch. I almost feel silly including this recipe since it's so variable

---

[66] Aimee Ryan, "Gut-Healing Vegetable Broth (And Why It's Better than Bone Broth), Wallflower Kitchen (Aug 18, 2016) https://wallflowerkitchen.com/gut-healing-vegetable-broth-better-bone-broth/

and so easy to make, but "frittata" may be a new term to some, so this should take the mystery out.

A frittata is essentially a lazy omelet. For a veggie frittata, instead of cooking the eggs and veggies separately, you sauté the vegetables (I often use broccoli, spinach, mushrooms, and onions). In a separate bowl, crack two eggs and beat them well, adding pepper and salt to taste. Then, while the veggies are tender and still hot on the stove, pour the eggs over and around them, tilting the pan for uniform cooking. After just a minute or two, pop the pan under the broiler to cook the top of the frittata. When it begins to brown, the frittata is done, and you can slide it out onto a plate and enjoy.

I tend to use well-seasoned cast-iron pans for all my frying and sauteing, and these can go right under the broiler as well. Tip: You can use four or five eggs and cut the frittata in two after cooking, saving half for another day.

Quiche muffins

I discovered this recipe when I tried my strictly keto experiment that lasted a couple of months. As a keto newbie, I bought a half-dozen keto cookbooks and found several recipes that we continue to use today. I especially enjoyed those by Cristina Curp and Maria Emmerich. I found the following recipe in Cristina Curp's *Made Whole* recipe book.

Makes six regular-size muffins or 12 mini muffins; prep time: 15 minutes; cook time: 35 minutes for mini muffins, 25 min for regular-size muffins.

Ingredients

- 4 slices bacon, diced
- 2 cups rainbow slaw or other shredded vegetables
- 1 tsp fine Himalayan salt, divided
- 5 large eggs
- ½ tsp ground black pepper
- ½ tsp dried Italian herb blend
- ½ cup full-fat coconut milk
- ¼ cup nutritional yeast

For the crust

- ¼ cup coconut flour
- 4-5 Tbsp flaxseed meal
- ¼ cup lard, unsalted butter or ghee, softened
- 1–3 Tbsp ice-cold water

1. Preheat the oven to 400 degrees. Line muffin tin with baking cups or use coconut oil spray. If you use baking cups, lightly grease them with coconut oil or avocado oil.
2. In a large skillet, cook the bacon over medium-high heat until crispy, stirring occasionally. Remove the bacon from the skillet and set it on a plate to cool, leaving the fat in the skillet. Add the rainbow slaw and ½ tsp of the salt to the skillet. Cover and cook for about 10 minutes, stirring occasionally.

3. While the slaw cooks, make the crust: Mix the coconut flour and flaxseed meal in a small bowl. Add the lard and use your fingertips to break it up until a crumbly dough forms. Add the water a tablespoon at a time, until the dough comes together and you can form it into a large ball. Cover the bowl and place it in the fridge.

4. By now, the slaw should be done. Remove it from the skillet and transfer it onto a plate with the bacon to cool.

5. In a large bowl, whisk together the eggs, remaining ½ tsp of salt, seasonings, and coconut milk. Add the nutritional yeast and whisk until well combined.

6. Remove the dough from the fridge. Break off ½-inch pieces and press them down into the bottom of the muffin cups, creating little crusts. Par-bake for 5 minutes.

7. While the crust is par-baking, mix the cooled saw and bacon into the egg mixture.

8. Remove the crusts from the oven and ladle the egg and slaw mixture into the muffin cups, filling them ¾ full. Bake for 15 minutes (mini muffins) or until the centers are set and the muffins are fluffy and golden. (I leave the regular size muffins in for 25 minutes and find that's just right.) Let cool 5 minutes before serving.

Store in an airtight container in the fridge for up to one week. To reheat, toast in a preheated 350-degree oven for 8–10 minutes.

One serving = one regular or two mini muffins

Calories: 155, fat: 12.5g, carbohydrates: 4.6 g., fiber: 2.3g, protein: 6.6 g.

Zoodles

Zoodles can be a one-ingredient recipe (spiralized zucchini), or for more interest, you can steam them, add butter, salt, pepper, and oregano. (You can do the same with pasta. I did this for my son and now he feels maltreated if I serve it any other way.)

Baked sweet potatoes

Sweet potatoes are more nutritious than white potatoes (for instance, they have a higher vitamin A content), and because they are lower on the glycemic index, they're less likely to cause your blood sugar to spike. I like to coat sweet potatoes in coconut oil, sprinkle them all over with Himalayan salt, and then poke them a few times with a fork to ensure they won't explode during cooking. I don't wrap them in foil when baking, which, combined with the salt, makes for a delicious crispy skin. I cook several at a time and use the leftovers to make an easy hash, chopping them up and adding sauteed vegetables, such as onion and bell peppers.

Minute English muffin

This recipe is from Maria Emmerich's cookbook, *Quick & Easy Ketogenic Cooking*. It takes longer than a minute, but it's pretty darn quick. If you're trying to go low carb and miss your bread, this is a great substitute, and it only has 3.3 carbs, 16.7g fat, 6.7g protein—a perfect ratio of 79% fat, 14% protein, and 7% carbs. It also contains

2g of fiber, so if you're counting "net carbs" as some people do, subtract fiber grams from carb grams to get 1.3 net carbs. I try to keep to 20 grams of carbs total when I'm being strictly keto, but see what works best for you.

Ingredients

- 1 tsp unsalted butter (I use salted, but whatever you have is fine) or coconut oil for greasing the ramekin (you can also use coconut oil spray or avocado oil spray)
- 1 large egg
- 2 tsp coconut flour
- Pinch of baking soda
- Pinch of fine sea salt
- 1 Tbsp grated parmesan cheese (optional; omit for dairy-free)
- 2 tsp coconut oil (for frying—optional cooking method)

1. Grease a 4-oz dessert ramekin with the butter or oil. Preheat toaster oven to 400 degrees if that's how you're cooking it.
2. In a small mixing bowl, mix the egg and coconut flour with a fork until well combined, then add the rest of the ingredients and stir to combine.
3. Place the dough in the greased ramekin. If you're using a microwave, cook on high for one minute. If you're using a toaster oven, cook for 12 minutes or until a toothpick comes out clean. (I like to add a sprinkle of sesame seeds on top of the muffin before baking. I also add some onion powder to the mix for flavor.)

4. Allow to cook for five minutes, then remove from the ramekin and allow to cool completely. For a muffin with crispy edges, slice the muffin in half and fry in the coconut oil (cut side down) over medium heat.

Pantry Staples

Stocking up on the right ingredients and jettisoning (or storing away) the wrong ones will make your fasting journey much easier.

Look for products without added sugar. This can sometimes be challenging because, in the US, we add it to so much, but it's worth looking for it! Tomato sauce, spaghetti sauce, and salad dressings can all be loaded with sugar if we're not careful in our shopping. For turkey bacon, look for the paleo version because regular turkey bacon often has added sugar.

Coconut flour and almond flour. These flours are lower in carbs and higher in nutritional value than wheat flour. Those who have trouble with gluten probably already know their benefits.

Avocado oil, coconut oil, and MCT oil. I use these oils for cooking because they have a higher burn threshold than olive oil. Vegetable oils, such as canola, safflower, corn, etc., should be avoided due to over-processing. Olive oil is great, and I use it all the time, but not for cooking. As mentioned, when you heat olive oil to its smoke point, the beneficial compounds in the oil begin to degrade, sometimes imparting a bitter flavor to food, and health-harming free radicals form. Save olive oil for cold uses, such as salad dressing. Some people don't like the idea of using coconut oil when they cook because they don't like coconut flavor (I happen to love coconut!).

But good news: refined coconut oil doesn't have a coconut flavor. It can be expensive in smaller amounts, but organic, non-GMO coconut oil is available in a large tub at the price clubs, and it will last forever.

I also use coconut oil for small burn and wound treatment, body moisturizer, hair smoother (a little goes a long way!), makeup removal, and oil pulling (the process of swishing oil through your mouth) for healthy gums and detoxification. Don't swallow if you oil pull, and don't spit it out into the drain. Spit it into a paper cup or tissue and dispose of it. Then rinse with Himalayan salt water, and spit that into the sink.

Filtered water. No, it's not a pantry staple, but since water is a big part of what you should be consuming every day (unless you're dry fasting), I'll tell you my water routine. For eight years or so, we've only used filtered water. Unless I'm somewhere where it's the only choice for hydration I avoid water bottles made of plastic. When plastic heats (as it can in warehouses in storage), chemicals can leach into the water. Instead, we use a water filtration system called Big Berkey, which makes 2.5 gallons at a time. It's serious stuff. I want the water we consume to be as pure as possible, so I even cook pasta, make coffee, and steam vegetables with it.

Coffee filters. And, speaking of coffee, if you use a coffee maker that requires a filter, be sure to use the unbleached kind. The white, bleached coffee filters can leach chemicals into your coffee. Our environment contains enough toxins, so the more we can reduce our toxic load, the happier our bodies will be.

Coconut flour tortillas. I found these recently, and my son (who is gluten-free) loves them. They don't have a coconut flavor and are more pliable (especially if you warm them first) for wrapping burritos, quesadillas, and enchiladas than some of the gluten-free flours out there.

Organic everything. I buy almost exclusively organic. Look around for alternatives to Whole Foods, which some call Whole Paycheck. When we lived on Maui, I found two great local markets that offered mostly organic produce, and they had great prices, especially for Maui. In Portland, we shop mostly at Natural Grocers, a store that tends to have much better prices than Whole Foods—but not for everything. Be sure to price compare. It's especially important to purchase organic versions of the fruits and veggies known as the Dirty Dozen because they have been found to have more pesticide residue than that found in other produce:

1. Strawberries
2. Spinach
3. Kale, collard, and mustard greens
4. Nectarines
5. Apples
6. Grapes (and by association, wine)
7. Cherries
8. Peaches
9. Pears
10. Bell and hot peppers

11. Celery
12. Tomatoes (and by association, tomato paste and tomato sauce)

Swerve. This is a natural sweetener, not bitter like stevia can be, and can be substituted 1:1 for recipes that call for sugar. It comes in granular and powdered varieties and is expensive.

Himalayan salt. There's very little reason to buy white table salt when pink Himalayan salt is easy to obtain and contains far more nutrients (and frankly tastes better) than white salt. It's available in fine, regular, and rock salt varieties, and the rock salt varieties often come with their own grinders. One reason cited for using table salt is its higher iodine content as compared to Himalayan salt. If iodine deficiency is a concern (often when thyroid issues are present), take that into consideration.

Freezer Items

- Bone broth (homemade or store-bought)
- Organic blueberries
- Cauliflower rice

Gadgets and Cookware

- Glass bowls with close-fitting plastic lids for storage
- Cast iron fry and sauté pans
- Galvanized aluminum saucepans

- A spiralizer for making zoodles (the small handheld ones are easier to clean and use, and are less expensive than the countertop versions)
- A good quality toaster oven

The toaster oven was a switch I made when living on Maui. It can get very warm there, and the idea of heating up our condo by turning on a huge oven (especially given that electricity is expensive there) made no sense to me. I purchased a Breville toaster oven, and we cook everything in that. It even fits a full-size pizza!

I sold the original Breville when we moved back to the mainland, but quickly bought another. A good quality toaster oven heats up faster and is much more convenient to use than a full-size oven. If you get one, you'll probably find yourself eating in more often and enjoying cooking more. We use our full-size oven only once or twice a year when we need more capacity. The rest of the time it serves as a cupboard for our pots and pans.

A FINAL THOUGHT

Expect Resistance

ALTHOUGH IT'S CERTAINLY NOT NEW, intermittent fasting has been having a moment for several years now, and as the buzz about it has risen, I've begun to see some negative articles warning about its dangers, predicting all kinds of maladies. This is only going to increase as more and more people discover its benefits and begin breaking the hamster wheel that has us paying for diets, programs, products, pharmaceuticals, and surgeries we no longer need—and that most of us never needed.

Fasting is a time-honored tradition in many religions that has been practiced for thousands of years with no one raising an eyebrow. That is, until it began reversing type 2 diabetes and helping people break free from the stranglehold of the weight-loss industry.

Fasting earns no one money (although it saves you plenty), therefore in the $79B weight loss industry, it's bound to become

Public Enemy Number One. They're either going to try to demonize it or monetize it. Don't listen, don't buy. If you have any doubt that you need to take what's said by "authoritative sources" with a grain of salt, then read the article "The Corruption of Evidence Based Medicine – Killing for Profit" on Dr. Fung's website, The Fasting Method.

But—What Will I Tell My Friends?

I recommend you don't tell your friends you're fasting, particularly not the ones who you know will give you grief about it. Or hand them this book or point them to Dr. Fung's books or YouTube videos if they have questions. Other authoritative sources are Dr. Eric Berg, Dr. Becky Gillaspy, and Dr. Mindy Pelz (Dr. Pelz has a series on YouTube on women's hormones and intermittent fasting).

It's hard for some people to imagine going without food for even a few hours. If you need to explain why you're not eating, simply state, "I'm sticking to a specific eating schedule for health reasons."

If You Decide Fasting Is Not For You

Even though fasting has significant health benefits, not everyone will be a fan. I will go weeks—even a couple of months—without fasting at all. I get busy, and food just seems like a good idea. But I know I can go back to it when I'm ready and mentally prepared.

If you've given fasting a good try and you don't feel it's right for you at this time, or you don't think you'll ever try it, don't sweat it. The whole idea of this book is you being in control of your own eating: when and what. Provided you have no serious health issues requiring you to fast, wait until you're ready. Fasting is yours to use or not when you want.

And if you do decide to fast and need motivation, here's another post from an intermittent fasting Facebook group. You can use this for any new healthy habit you're trying to create, substituting the appropriate words.

Fasting is hard. Being unhealthy is hard. Pick your hard.

BONUS: AFFIRMATIONS

Affirmations for Your Intermittent Fasting Journey

IF YOU'VE TRIED AFFIRMATIONS in the past and they didn't really work for you, I have a couple of tips that may help. First, only choose affirmations you can believe. Never lie to yourself. Try each of the following affirmations and see which feel true to you. Work with those and revisit the others as you grow stronger in your belief in yourself.

The other tip is that simply saying the affirmation is not enough. *The Spontaneous Healing of Belief* is a wonderful book by Gregg Braden, who studies the wisdom of indigenous people. Braden says that feeling affirmations, rather than just saying or writing them, is what gives them their power. He learned this when visiting an 800-

year-old monastery in Tibet. The monks there toned and chanted for 14–16 hours a day, using bells, bowls, gongs, chimes, mudras, and mantras. Through a translator, Braden asked the abbot, "When we see you doing your prayers like that, what are you really doing? What is happening to you on the inside?" The abbot answered, "You have never seen our prayers because a prayer cannot be seen. What you have seen is what we do to create the feeling in our bodies. Feeling is the prayer."

Other tips on affirmations may be found in Jack Canfield's bestseller, *The Success Principles: How to Get from Where You Are to Where You Want to Be*. Here are three he suggests:

1. Start with the word "I am." It's been said that whatever follows those words is your belief in yourself. Never follow those words with negative thoughts. Per Canfield, these are "the two most powerful words in the language. The subconscious takes any sentence that starts with the word I am and interprets it as a command—a directive to make it happen."[67]
2. Use the present tense. Describe what you want as if you already have it; it's already accomplished.
3. State it in the positive. Our subconscious doesn't know how to interpret "not." Try this: Don't think of an elephant. What image popped into your head? Exactly.

---

[67] Jack Canfield, *The Success Principles*, p. 75–80. Collins, 2007.

Before you start with the affirmations, which you should try to do at least three times a day—on waking, during a quiet spot in your day, and before bed—take three deep cleansing breaths.

Imagine that you are a tall tree with thick roots that connect deep into Mother Earth. You are strong and balanced. You are safe. You are powerful.

- I am strong and balanced.
- I am a goddess, a divine being of love and light.
- I am courageous and brimming with energy.
- I am powerful.
- My body is perfect and whole as it is right now.
- I make positive choices for my health, my vitality, and my spirit.
- I am ready to change my life for the better.
- I choose to live my best life now.
- My intuition is always on my side. I trust it to guide me wisely.
- My healing is already in process.
- My body is worthy of great care.
- My body is wise. It knows what to do.
- I am connected to the silent, powerful intelligence of my body.
- Fasting refreshes and restores my body.
- Every day I fast, I lose excess fat, becoming leaner and stronger.

- My body is strong and active.
- My body properly digests the food I eat.
- I find it easy to drink enough water.
- I know how to make healthy choices and I have a healthy relationship with food.
- The food I eat keeps me energized and satisfied.
- Fasting detoxes my entire body from the inside out.
- I know how to work with my body for optimum health.
- My body loves and protects me. Eating healthy food is my way of loving and protecting my body.
- My mind is clear and focused.
- I can achieve more than I ever thought possible.
- I am capable of fasting when I choose.
- I radiate good health.
- All my actions, food, and thoughts support the wellbeing of my body, mind, and spirit.
- I am living my ideal life.
- Fasting refreshes and restores my body.
- I am excited about who I'm becoming as I step more and more into my power every day.
- I fulfill the promises I make to myself and others.
- Fasting strengthens my will to achieve optimum health.
- I am always in control of what I eat.
- I am filled with energy.
- I speak kindly to myself.
- I grow stronger every day.

- My health and happiness are my greatest accomplishments.
- I have all the strength I need to accomplish my goals.
- My body is releasing toxins and purifying itself.
- I grow younger and more vibrant every day.
- Fasting energizes me and makes me feel alive.
- When I fast, I am alert, energetic, and focused.
- I am successful in everything I do.
- Fasting gives me more time to do what I enjoy each day.
- I am unstoppable.
- I have all the strength I need to accomplish my goals.
- I choose a healthier, happier me.
- Fasting allows me to rest and rejuvenate.
- I am mentally, spiritually, and emotionally clear.
- Every cell in my body radiates happiness.
- Fasting releases endorphins, and I feel very happy.
- My body is releasing old and damaged cells.
- My brain is becoming more and more resistant to stress.
- My body is becoming a fat-burning machine.
- I am reclaiming my health and wellbeing.
- I am in tune with and love my body.
- I love water. It quenches my thirst and purifies my body.
- Fasting clears my mind, and I am more energetic, productive, happy, and centered.

Acknowledgments

FIRST AND FOREMOST, I owe a great debt to **Ellen Barski**, who first told me about the 5/2 method and intermittent fasting; she also provided encouragement and early feedback on this book.

I also owe my gratitude to my mastermind group. Members include **Audrey Sweet**, **Sahara Miller**, and **Sara Pehrsson**. All were very supportive of the book concept and provided great feedback through every phase. If you don't know what a mastermind group is, please check out my book *How to Create a Mastermind Group: The Power Hour Ticket to Everything You've Ever Wanted,* which I authored under a pen name, Celeste Maxwell. A mastermind really is a game changer.

My gratitude also goes to **Cheryl Hoeppner**, editor extraordinaire. Cheryl is a generous and diplomatic editor who hardly ever laughs at my gaffes, such as "stationery bike." She edited the first final draft, but much to my surprise, I wasn't finished yet, and have made changes since. So, if you find any gaffes, they're not Cheryl's fault.

Thank you also to **Kelly Seibert**, who never fails to make me think that I know what I'm doing and who gave me what may be my favorite gift ever, a coffee mug that reads "This is what a published author looks like." *Kelly, you're next.*

To my sons, **Max** and **Sam**, the reason for everything. And to all my friends and family who provide support, encouragement, and beta reviews, you rock, and I wouldn't want to do this without you.

And last, but not least, I am indebted to **Dr. Jason Fung** for his pioneering work with fasting and its therapeutic application for reversing obesity and type 2 diabetes. We need more doctors like him who not only believe what's before their very eyes (even if it doesn't agree with prevailing theories) but are also willing to dig for better answers and then share what they've learned with the masses. I've recommended three of his books for further reading.

To You, Goddess

I hope this book has in some small way shown you that you are and always will be the driving force for change in your life and that the answers were never "out there" but are and always will be inside of you. I hope you now have the tools you've been looking for to enable you to work with your body for optimal health.

I wish I could transport myself from these pages, look into your eyes, and tell you what an amazing, rare, gifted, talented, lovable, powerful, strong, beautiful person you are. I wish I could say that right to your face so you could see that I mean it. Please believe this: We need you. There will never be another you in all the eons, for all time. And no matter what size, shape, color, nationality, orientation, pronoun, political affiliation, education, income level, background, or religion you have, you are a gift to the world.

You are a goddess. You are bigger than dieting and you have more important things to do with your life than obsess about numbers on a scale. Now … let's go kick some ass.

For Further Reading

Frozen Assets: How to Cook for a Day and Eat for a Month, by Deborah Taylor-Hough, Champion Press, 1999.

How to Live Longer and Feel Better, by Linus Pauling, Oregon State University Press, 2006.

Keto Restaurant Favorites: More than 1785 Tasty Classic Recipes Made Fast, Fresh, and Healthy, by Maria Emmerich, Victory Belt Publishing, 2017.

Made Whole: More Than 145 Anti-Inflammatory Keto-Paleo Recipes to Nourish You from the Inside Out, by Cristina Curp, Victory Belt Publishing, 2018.

Quick and Easy Ketogenic Cooking: Time-Saving Paelo Recipes and Meal Plans to Improve Your Health and Help You Lose Weight, by Maria Emmerich, Victory Belt Publishing, 2016.

The Case Against Sugar by Gary Taubes, Knopf (2016)

The Complete Guide to Intermittent Fasting: Heal Your Body Through Intermittent, Alternate-Day, and Extended Fasting, by Jason Fung, MD, Victoria Belt Publishing, 2016.

The Diabetes Code: Prevent and Reverse Type 2 Diabetes Naturally (The Wellness Code Book Two) (The Code Series, 2), Jason Fung, MD, Graystone Books, 2018.

The Obesity Code: Unlocking the Secrets of Weight Loss: Why Intermittent Fasting Is the Key to Controlling Your Weight, by Jason Fung, MD, Graystone Books, 2016.

The Spontaneous Healing of Belief: Shattering the Paradigm of False Limits, by Gregg Braden, Hay House Inc., 2008.

The Success Principles: How to Get from Where You Are to Where You Want to Be, by Jack Canfield, HarperCollins, 2005.

Wheat Belly, by William Davis, MD, Rodale Books, 2011.

Why We Sleep: Unlocking the Power of Sleep and Dreams, by Matthew Walker, PhD, Scribner, 2017.

Younger Next Year: Live Strong, Fit, Sexy, and Smart—Until You're 80 and Beyond, by Chris Crowley and Henry S. Lodge, MD, Workman Publishing Company, 2019.

About the Author

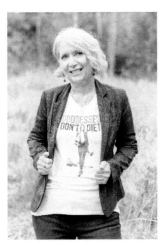

Yvonne Aileen is a researcher and author who practices intermittent fasting for weight control and health benefits.

She lives in a suburb of Portland, Oregon with her sons Max and Sam.

A Note from the Publisher

If you enjoyed this book, please leave a review on the site of your favorite bookseller. This helps other goddesses find it. *Thank you.*

Made in United States
Cleveland, OH
17 July 2025